# Intermittent Fasting & Keto

# After 50

## *This Book Includes 2 Manuscripts:*

## *Two Complete Guides To Restart Metabolism and Boost Energy for Women and Men Over 50 | 2 Books in 1 |*

## Michelle Clarity

# Table of Contents

**Conclusion 340**

# KETO AFTER 50

*RESTART YOUR METABOLISM AND BOOST YOUR ENERGY; THE ULTIMATE 2020 GUIDE TO KETOGENIC DIET FOR SENIORS OVER 50 | LOSE WEIGHT & CUT CHOLESTEROL IN A HEALTHY WAY |*

# Introduction

Before starting any diet, it is crucial you understand the history behind it. As you well know, there are many diets on the market in the modern age. The right question you need to ask for yourself is, Is the Ketogenic Diet right for you? Luckily for all of us, the Ketogenic Diet can help a wide range of individuals, whether you are young, older, or somewhere in between!

## History of the Ketogenic Diet

The Ketogenic Diet first began in the 1920s and 30s. Initially, it was a popular therapy for individuals who had epilepsy. At the very beginning, the Ketogenic Diet was first developed to provide an alternative to fasting, which also worked well for epilepsy therapy.

While the diet did work for a while for these patients, it was eventually abandoned when modern medicine came around and was able to help a majority of patients with their symptoms. However, there were still approximately 30% of patients where the medication did not work, and the diet was re-introduced to help these individuals.

In 1921, it was an endocrinologist known as Rollin Woodyatt that was one of the first to notice the three water-soluble compounds that are produced in the liver when we are starved from carbohydrates. These three compounds are what we now know as ketone bodies. It was at this point, an individual from the Mayo

Clinic known as Russel Wilder would call this "starvation from carbohydrates" as the Ketogenic Diet!

It is imperative to note that the ketogenic diet for people in their 30s is different from those in their 50s. The main difference is in the amount of energy required to do various activities. In your younger years, you will need more energy to allow you to carry out your activities easily. There is solid evidence that a ketogenic diet can reduced seizures. Since it has neuroprotective features, your brain cells will be replenished, and you will not experience memory loss quickly. Some studies suggest that a ketogenic diet can help in preventing disorders such as Alzheimer's, sleep disorders, autism, and Parkinson's disease. Weight loss is the most important aspect of a ketogenic diet, and you can easily lose weight with the ketogenic diet. It will help in improving blood sugar levels as well as rejuvenating your brain cells as well as give you a feel-good mood.

Although the diet is solely based on fats and proteins, you should try and take fats and proteins that are healthy. Avoid processed salty foods as well as fats with low-density lipoproteins. Eating healthy is the first way of building a better immune system and a better mood throughout the day. Choose the ketogenic diet and enjoy the benefits that come with it.

A ketogenic diet provides your body with premium fuel, which is fat, and it makes you feel fitter, stronger, and younger. You can achieve all this by following a diet that will burn away excess fat and take your body and health to a whole new level. So why is the ketogenic diet the most preferred type of diet for people after 50?

A ketogenic diet is considered as a miracle diet because it will turn around your health and allow your cells to rejuvenate quickly. The body has different metabolic pathways that are essential in the production of energy. However, some are used more than others because of cellular preference. The main source of energy in the body is usually glucose, and this is the simplest form of sugar.

Most of the sugar that we consume is a pure form of glucose; on the other hand, some of the carbohydrates can be broken down into glucose. When the body runs low on glucose, it can break down fats into energy, and this is a process called gluconeogenesis. Besides, the body can run on other energy sources such as free fatty acids and ketones. However, it is important to note that the body will only run on alternative sources of energy once glucose is depleted in the system. The depletion of glucose in the body usually results from fasting or eating a diet that is low in carbohydrates.

The glucose depletion process can take anywhere from 24 to 36 hours, although this process can be sped up by carrying out various forms of exercises. As the glucose reserves get depleted, the body will compensate for the energy needs by burning free fatty acids.

As the diet continues to grow in popularity, there is more research being performed on the Ketogenic Diet by the day! With science-backed evidence, you can follow the diet and know for a fact that it is going to work.

Welcome to your first Ketogenic Diet Science lesson! One of the best parts of the Ketogenic Diet is the fact that it is based around a natural process that your body already has! The key to success is fueling your body correctly instead of stuffing it with overly-processed junk. In this guide, you will learn everything you need to know from what to eat when to eat and how to get into the best shape of your life!

# Chapter 1: What is Ketogenic

Keto, short for ketogenic, is a form of diet that primarily focuses on cutting down carbs and increasing the protein intake of a person. The idea is that you cut back and remove all the easy-to-digest carbs from your regular intake such as sugar, white bread, sodas, and so on. In return, you are left with a healthy dose of good fats, a sufficient amount of protein, and a much lower amount of carbohydrates.

This is a general description of what a keto diet does, but that alone is not sufficient to base a decision upon. I know, I was certainly attracted by the general idea and how it sounded, but I needed more than just a line or two about what keto does. I needed to know exactly what goes on within our body and how keto can fit the picture, especially for people who have a few pounds popping out of proportion and age that is rapidly approaching the 60 years mark.

## The Science Behind It

The idea behind most diets remains the same. One needs to reduce the amount of carbs intake in a day and the weight should fall. The problem is that most diets require you to stop eating or skip meals to bring the carb level down. For a very long time, I had wondered if there was any other way to address this issue.

Certainly, the idea of losing weight is appealing. It is a motivator that pushes us to stop eating and force our body to start converting stored fats into fuel to burn. Sounds good, but the hunger that comes in is a killer.

The catch behind cutting down on carbs is simple, it makes your body run low on glucose. When that happens, the state of ketosis is in effect. This is where ketones come to the rescue as your body's natural fuel backup. Here's a little fact: we only ever enter into the state of ketosis if we starve ourselves for a few days, not just overnight or by skipping a meal. That, then, is quite a tough prospect.

In keto, things work a little differently, and fortunately a little more friendly. The principle remains the same, you force your body to switch the ketosis mode on, but instead of starving yourself for food, you just cut down the amount of carbs while continuing to consume other nutrients. Slice it anyway you like, but this is genuinely more interesting and easier to do.

By removing all sorts of carbs, including but not limited to complex carbs, starches, and refined carbs, we will force our body to lose glucose and be left with no other source to acquire more. This will then switch our body into ketosis to allow ketones to make their way to the brain and resume normal functions. Our brain requires either glucose or ketones to function, and through ketosis, it gets the necessary supply.

What follows afterwards is a continuous process of our body breaking down fats into ketones regardless of how much protein or fat you consume. The result is a satisfied hunger and weight loss that changes everything for you; a feat many diets cannot deliver.

The world has been taken by storm at just how easy this diet can be and how it can deliver magnificent results. Keto diets are almost for everyone who are suffering from weight issues and are unable to lose their extra pounds. Through careful selection of food and monitoring the intake the keto way, you should be able to see the results rather quickly.

It goes without saying that for a weight loss solution, keto is looking up like a perfect contender. Not only do you not need to give up eating, but you can enjoy scrumptious meals while losing your weight through techniques which otherwise would require you to starve to near death. In addition to these facts, most keto recipes are extremely easy to cook, and most of them taste equally delicious. This means you do not have to rely on bitter tasting drinks, weird looking food, or lack thereof.

Keto is quite popular, and for a very good reason. It genuinely promotes healthy eating without pushing anyone into a state of jeopardy. The success rate of keto is rather high. While there are no specific numbers to suggest the exact rate, it is only fair to state that those who have the will to change their lifestyle and are okay adjusting to new eating habits, almost every one of them will make it through as a success story.

## What is Ketosis?

Ketosis is a metabolic state where the body is efficiently using fat for energy. In a regular diet, carbohydrates produce glucose, which is used to provide energy. Glucose is stored in the body in fat cells that travel via the bloodstream. People gain weight when there is more fat stored than being used as energy.

Glucose is formed through the consumption of sugar and starch. Namely carbohydrates. The sugars may be in the form of natural sugars from fruit or milk, or they may be formed from processed sugar. Starches like pasta, rice or starchy vegetables like potatoes and corn, form glucose as well. The body breaks down the sugars from these foods into glucose. Glucose and insulin combined to help to carry glucose into the bloodstream so the body can use glucose as energy. The glucose that is not used is stored in the liver and muscles.

In order for the body to supply ketones for use as fuel, the body must use up all the reserves of glucose. In order to do this, there must be a condition of the body of starvation low carbohydrates, passing, or strenuous exercise. A very low carb diet, the production of ketones what her to feel the body and brain.

## Why Is It Important for People Over 50?

Now comes the interesting part. I am sure you have been wondering how it will help you, a person who is 50 years or more in age, and why is it so important, right? Do not worry as I shall provide you with an answer that satisfies both questions.

A few minutes ago, we read how keto diet pushes our body into ketosis; a state where ketones take over the role of glucose. That may sound good for younger people than you, but the fact is that it is actually a better fit for someone your age. Why, I hear you ask?

As you grow in age, the body's natural fat burning ability reduces. When that happens, your body stops receiving a healthy dose of nutrients properly, which is why you will develop diseases and ailments. With the keto diet, you are pushing the body into ketosis and bypassing the need to worry about your body's ability to burn fat. Once in ketosis, your body will now burn fat forcefully for survival.

Once more, your system will now start to regain strength. An even better aspect that follows is your insulin level because it drops. If you are someone diagnosed with diseases such as type 2 diabetes and others, the drop in insulin might even reverse the effects and eliminate the diseases from your body altogether.

There are studies underway, and most of them suggest that keto diet is far more beneficial to those above 50 than it is for those under this age bracket. A quick search on Google and you are immediately overwhelmed with over 93 million results, most of which explain the benefits of the keto diet for people above 50. That is a staggering number for a diet plan that has only been around a few years.

It is also important to highlight that as we get older, we start losing more than just the ability to burn fat. During this phase of our life, once we hit around 50 years of age, we come across various obstacles, some chronic in nature, which transpire only because our body is no longer able to function at rates like it did when we were young. Ketogenic diets help us regain that edge and feel energized from within.

There are hundreds of thousands of stories, all pointing out how this revolutionary diet is especially helpful for older adults and the elderly. It is therefore a no-brainer for people above 50 who have spent ages trying to search for a healthy lifestyle choice of diet. With such a high success rate, there is no harm in trying, right?

Before the keto phenomenon, there was the Atkins diet. The Atkins diet was also a low carb diet, just like its keto counterpart. This form of diet also became a huge hit with the masses. However, unlike keto, the Atkins diet provided weight loss while putting a person through constant hunger. Keto, on the other hand, takes away that element, and it does that using ketosis.

Constant exposure to ketosis reduces appetite, hence taking away the biggest hurdle in most diets. The Atkins diet failed to address that front, which is why it was more of a hit and miss. However, credit where it is due, the Atkins diet did garner quite a bit of fame. However, since the inception of keto, things have changed dramatically.

A study was conducted where 34 overweight adults were monitored and observed for 12 months. All of them were put on keto diets. The end result showed that participants had lower HgbA1c (hemoglobin A1c) levels, experienced significant weight loss, and were more likely to completely discontinue their medications for diabetes.

All in all, the keto diet is shaping up to be quite a promising candidate for older adults. Not only will this diet allow us to lead a healthier lifestyle, but it will also curb our ailments and ensure high energy around the clock. That is quite the resume for a diet, and one that now seems too attractive to pass up. This is the point where I made up my mind and decided to give the keto diet a go, and I recommend the same to you.

Whether you are a man or a woman, if you have put on weight, or you are suffering from ailments like type 2 diabetes, consider this as your ticket to a care-free world where you will lead a healthy life and rise out of the ailments eventually.

Keto has been producing results which has attracted the top minds and researchers for a fairly long time. Considering the unique nature of this lifestyle of eating, the results have been rather encouraging.

## Body Changes after 50

We are all getting older. Of course, you are no exception. This process is inevitable, and it makes your life saturated in all aspects. When you're 50-something, you gain wisdom and life experience, you build meaningful relationships and mental strength. But don't forget that not only internal changes occur after age 50. Your body also changes and you need to prepare for that.

### Your Metabolic Rate Slows Down

When you have reached the age of 50, your body starts digesting food in a different way as a result of a decreased metabolic rate. Chemical reactions inside your body that are responsible for burning the calories you consume become slower. It is entirely normal and doesn't mean that you should eat less or reduce the portion sizes on your plate. This peculiarity implies that you should pay more attention to your meal plan as you age and choose the food that fits best for your nutritional needs as well as goals.

### Your Muscle Power Decreases

At the old age, muscle mass and, therefore, strength reduces. Physical inactivity and an unhealthy diet are the leading causes of this negative change in a 50-something-year-old's body. But it is in your power to prevent this change.

### Your Bones Become More Brittle

When it comes to the bones, you gotta understand that their condition is also more likely to change after 50. Hormonal imbalance, and loss of calcium and other crucial minerals in bones result in low bone density and a higher risk of injury.

### Your Excess Weight Increases

Perhaps the only thing that rises with age is the figure on your scales. As you get older, you can experience disappointing changes in your body. In most cases, you notice them when looking in the mirror and weighing yourself. Extra pounds are a real problem for people who are over 50 and the most unpleasant task is getting rid of this dead weight. Well, this is one more reason why you need to focus on the Keto diet and look closely at all the benefits of this low-carb eating plan for older people.

# Benefits of the Keto Diet for People over 50

If you're a person who's already celebrated your 50th birthday, that doesn't mean that your life becomes dull from here on, and you don't know how to spend your free time. Quite the opposite! You may often feel time-crunch because of work, family, and generally because of various life situations. Actually, it can be quite difficult to make time for yourself and, moreover, finding time to plan a healthy diet is more likely to be last on the list of your priorities. However, you can change your attitude towards your nutritional needs and move them to the top of that list when you find out all the benefits of a low-carb, high-fat diet for older people.

- Improved Physical and Mental Health

With ageing you might notice an energy level drop due to different environmental and biological reasons. If you want to feel happy, active, and dynamic, pay closer attention to the Keto diet. Remember, reducing your carbohydrate intake usually leads to increasing your vital forces. When you start consuming a lower number of carbs, the body has to burn more fat to fuel itself. This process causes fat synthesis and ketone production, i.e. breaking down accumulated fat for energy. In such a way, the low-carbohydrate diet can stimulate brainpower and positive changes in cognition (like improving memory and concentration).

- Faster Metabolism

Older people have a slower metabolism. But thanks to the Keto diet, this problem can be solved. Excluding carb intake from your diet plan can help you to maintain healthy levels of blood sugar and, as a result, rev up your metabolism.

- Weight-Shedding

It is no big secret that as a person gets older, shedding weight gets harder. People after 50 face the challenge of weight-loss for a variety of reasons (from increasing levels of stress, slower metabolic rate to rapid muscle loss). The struggle with excess weight may take a lot of time and effort for people over the age of 50. But there is a way out, and it is called the Keto diet.

This peculiar diet is highly effective for losing weight because it boosts the metabolism of fat, and the body itself starts shedding stored fat. As an added bonus, people who stick to the Keto diet get a reduced appetite, which helps to prevent over-eating and, thus, quicker weight loss. Unlike many low-fat diets, the Ketogenic one doesn't recommend you to track your calories or eat less. There's no need for that! Keto usually leaves you feeling full and satisfied after a meal.

- Better Sleep

At an old age, people tend to have trouble sleeping. A lot of people over 50 experience such sleep disorders as insomnia, sleep apnea, restless leg syndrome, and sleepwalking. People aged 50 and over should know that a long-term Ketogenic diet can have a positive impact on sleep. A significant reduction in carb intake and, at the same time, a substantial increase in fat intake create favorable conditions for a night of deeper sleep, eliminate certain sleep disturbance triggers, and make a person more energetic when the sun is up.

- Protection from Age-Related Diseases

According to various scientific studies, the Keto diet can reduce the risks for specific age-related diseases, such as diabetes, different kinds of cancer, cardiovascular diseases, mental disorders, Parkinson's Disease, multiple sclerosis, and fatty liver disease.

# Chapter 2: Keto for Women Over 50

For married couples looking to improve their lifestyle, continue to read on.

Women—we go through so much in life, don't we? From growing up, discovering the joys of life, pursuing a promising career, becoming a mother; there is so much that changes within such a short span of time.

While that is a part of life, what anyone would genuinely try and avoid would be the part where we put on excessive weight that we carry around like an unneeded luggage. It is embarrassing, it is distracting, and it is causing quite a few internal issues as well.

If you thought the biggest hurdle you will face when you hit 50 is a big belly, think again. This isn't the only problem we face. While there are those who would say that having a generous belly is the biggest problem, I firmly believe that there are more serious issues to worry about than that. When it comes to women, well things aren't looking good.

Our bodies, since birth, continuously undergo changes. Most of these changes do not harm us and are only natural. However, once we enter into our 50s, things are a lot different. Now, any changes within our body will directly affect how we perform, operate and work. If we were to keep these changes unchecked and pay no close attention, things would take a turn for the worse.

Most of these issues will remain the same for men as well, however, due to the chemistry of our bodies and differences, both internal and external, both would end up facing a variety of issues exclusive to their gender.

There are a few ways we can avoid these issues. Some of these ways require you to go back in time and start working out from a very young age, control your diet, and change your habits. Obviously, that is the stuff of science fiction and hence is out of the equation.

Other ways would include visiting a doctor and getting pills and energy boosters to help us feel better while taking more pills to fight off diabetes, high blood pressure, and other health issues. This way is not just hectic but far too complicated as well.

For a very long time, the only other way was to avoid worrying too much and hope that life would fix issues itself, and that never ended well for many. People were then left with a worry and a gap that nothing was able to fill. In comes ketogenic diet.

Call it a need of the hour, a savior in disguise or anything you like, the fact remains that this is proving to be a popular option that is not only delivering results but is also helping millions to maintain a healthy lifestyle and reverse some of the damage their bodies have suffered.

Numerous studies have gone on to support the idea that keto diets are far more effective for the older men and women compared to the younger folks. With so much to look forward to and so little to sacrifice, it does make sense to state that keto is essentially becoming your permanent way of life once you hit 50, but why is that? Why is it that me and so many others are proclaiming keto as an important lifestyle choice for women above 50? The answer to this involves some explanation, but I will do my best to do just that!

## Keto: The Need of the Hour

Calling something the need of the hour is quite a statement. Anyone to claim something being so important must have sufficient material and facts to back such a claim with. While I have provided what exactly keto does, there is much to be learned and explored of just why keto is important for women over the age of 50.

So far, we have learned that women over 50 would face issues like:

- Being overweight
- Running low on energy
- Feeling drowsy and lethargic all the time
- Unable to focus on task
- Glucose levels going haywire
- Blood pressure issues

These are the most common ones but dig a little deeper and you quickly realize that these are just the tip of the iceberg that lies hidden in plain sight.

Menopause

There comes an age in a woman's life where her menstrual cycle will finally end. This is a phase that means your ovaries stop releasing eggs, better known as ovulation, and therefore menstruation ends. This condition is generally observed in women above the age of 40. There is no defined age that shows when a woman can expect menopause.

There are times where women may experience menopause prematurely as well. This happens if a woman has undergone surgeries like hysterectomy (surgery that involves removal of ovaries). It can also happen from any injuries that may have caused damage to the ovaries. If this happens before the age of 40, it is classified as premature menopause.

Menopause, as harmless as it sounds, can be quite a troubling phase for women. The hot flashes you experience will keep you up at night, with an elevated heartbeat. The constant feeling of being irritated and a clear downfall in your sex life can contribute greatly towards you feeling more and more grumpy.

Menopause takes a toll on your hormonal balance and the newly developed imbalance then pushes your body to gain massive weight, experience mood swings like never before and a libido that is crashing faster than you can imagine.

If you think this is bad, here are some other issues that menopause can lead to:

- Chronic stress
- Anxiety
- Insulin spike

- Type 2 Diabetes
- Heart Diseases
- Polycystic ovary syndrome (PCOS)

The overall picture, then, is grim! Fortunately, a difference of lifestyle and a carefully thought-out diet plan can change all that for you. I am not saying it happens overnight or within a week, but the profound impacts are felt rather quick. In the longer run, keto will rescue you and your body from impending doom and allow you to lead a life without worrying about keeping a glucose monitor or any of the typical health-related equipment near you.

The keto diet, while there are many classes of it, helps your hormones to remain in shape and balanced. This means that you do not have to worry about the insulin or any other hormones, hence minimizing the hot flashes and other symptoms. Even if they occur, they will be minor and far less painful.

Moreover, the keto diet jump-starts your sex drive. The fat-rich diet improves fat-soluble vitamin absorption. Not to forget it especially helps with vitamin D, a vital piece that goes missing with age. All in all, this provides all the drive you need to have intimate moments even in your fifties.

### Heart Diseases

Keto diets help women over 50 to shed those extra pounds. Reducing any amount of weight greatly reduces the chances of a heart attack or any other heart complications. Through the carefully selected diet routine, not only are you losing weight and enjoying scrumptious meals, but you are significantly boosting your heart's health and reviving yourself from the otherwise dull state that you may have been in before.

## Diabetes Control

Needless to say, the careful selection of ingredients, when cooked together, provide rich nutrients, free from any processed or harmful contents such as sugar. Add to that the fact that keto automatically controls your insulin levels. The result is a glucose level that is always under control and continued control would lead to a day where you will say goodbye to the medications you might be taking for diabetes.

## And so Much More!

By taking up the challenge and adapting the keto way, you are ensuring yourself one of the safest journeys into the older years, if not the safest of the lot. Sure, there will be days where you may miss a food or two, but that craving will be overshadowed by the benefits the keto diet will bring for you.

With the help of the keto diet, you can expect a few more benefits such as:

- Improved and stable blood pressure levels
- A deeper sleep for those suffering from insomnia
- Improved kidney function
- More energy that lasts all day
- Improved bodily functions

## All Set to Begin?

Great! Let me be the first one to let you know that you are not too late to start. The fact is, no one is ever too late to change their eating, sleeping, and working habits. All it takes is a spark of motivation, and if you are reading this line, you already have that spark. All you need now is to grab a pen and a paper to note down some fine recipes and jot down the things you need and the things you should avoid. Better yet, maintain a little diary or a notebook which you can refer to whenever you wish.

# Chapter 3: Keto for Men Over 50

Men—much like us women, you also go through quite a lot of internal and external changes. These include but are not limited to physical changes, habitual changes, and so on. While the chemistry inside the body of both remains broadly the same, whether young or old, there are things which men are more likely to develop or lose than women. These include some diseases, ailments, infections, habitual changes, and disorders. The worst news is, it happens as soon as you cross 45 years of age. That means you are at least five years late already, or at least that is what you think.

I was discussing about how a woman experiences changes within herself once she is 50 and up, I mentioned that it is never too late to begin your journey and pick up your very first keto routine. All it takes is a mind that is poised, a will that is evident, and a clear goal in sight. That is quite literally it.

However, unlike most diets which you can begin right away, there are a few things I should point out which men should keep an eye out for. Consider these as soft reminders or suggestions before you take up the keto challenge.

- **Keto diet is a lifestyle**: It is not a diet that you do for a few weeks and then resume your normal food and carb intake. This is a proper lifestyle that you will need to adopt and live with. As long as you continue abiding by its rules, you will continue to enjoy the benefits it has to offer.

- **Keto is not only meant for women**: There are those who actually believe that keto was designed specifically for women. I am here to set things right and let you know that keto is for both men and women.

- **Keto does not require you to cut down on your eating habits**: Not at all. With that said though, it does make you modify those habits by changing what you consume instead of how much you consume.

- **Keto food items may pose a risk to people with special medical conditions**: It is something that most websites, blogs, and articles fail to mention. If you suffer from issues like high cholesterol, be sure to do a bit of research regarding what you can use instead of a specific ingredient.

With that said, let us get down to details and find out just why keto is so important for men who are 50 years old and above.

## 50 Marks the Start of Troubles

Well, in all fairness, troubles for men may start a little sooner than that, but the reason I said that is because some of these troubles, such as diseases or issues related to obesity and weight gain, take some time to manifest themselves. It is usually around the 50-year mark where these issues come up almost immediately.

Now that you are within this age group, and are nearing your retirement age, there are so many things which can cause you to lose your patience, your focus, and depreciate your health as well. The biggest of these would be stress; the stress of not knowing what you will do once you have retired.

This stress can cause you to have insomnia, a massive eating disorder, and ultimately a body that is quickly running out of shape. With each passing year, you are incurring extra expenses upon yourself and trying to find a shirt and trousers that fits your new size. I completely understand that none of us, men or women, like to see that.

Stress is just the start of things; I haven't even begun to point out the medical issues a man's body can develop and be bombarded with. To give you an idea of what a 50-year-old male faces who is not observing any kind of diet, here is a list to digest:

- Anxiety

- Depression

- Uncontrollable blood pressure levels

- Diminishing sex drive

- Increased laziness

- Lack of energy

- Fluctuating insulin levels

Think about it, do any of these really sound the sort of issues you would be okay to face in such an age? Certainly, you need some form of assistance that can help you boost your morale, your spirits, and allow you to control life the way you had always done so.

"Exercise is the answer!" Well, yes and no.

You see, while exercise provides you with the muscular strength and some really good benefits, it is still not the ideal way to cut down on those extra pounds, nor will it allow you to control other bodily disorders. All exercise can do is to keep your body in shape physically. That is all there is to it. There is a simple reason for that.

Exercises are designed to utilize your body's energy and use it to carry out difficult tasks which, as a result, promote more strength and growth of muscles and mass. The keyword to focus here is "energy" and that is exactly where a diet comes in. In this case, we will be focusing on possibly the best diet of them all: keto.

The good news is that by combining your love of keto and exercise, you end up with the perfect duo that is always ready to complement each other. While they do that, you, the actual end-user, gets to enjoy a perfectly healthy lifestyle that is free from any harmful carbs or other nutrients.

For men over the age of 50, it is very much important to remain in good shape. This is something you would want to do as it allows you to carry out more tasks relatively easy and keeps you active throughout the day. But wait, there is more to keto than just that.

Through adopting a keto diet plan for your meals, and adding exercise to that, you are most likely to lead a longer life. Why do I say this? If you haven't noticed already, the keto diet comes with quite a lot of benefits.

The keto diet helps you to improve your blood sugar levels. This eliminates quite a lot of issues such as type 2 diabetes. Additionally, the keto plan helps you in keeping carbs at bay. This in return pushes your body to absorb fats as fuel instead. By doing so, your body will start to burn fats quicker than usual, and that is some good news for everyone.

As you grow old, some functions fade out while others slow down to a snail's pace. An example of the latter is the rate at which our body burns fat now versus how it used to burn fat when you were younger. There is a significant difference, and with keto you can recover that ability fairly easy as it trains your body to switch into ketosis mode.

This new change within your body would then make room for more energy. The more energy you have, the better you can work, focus, and carry out tasks. Finally, the keto diet never asks you to stop eating, and that means you always have a healthy meal waiting for you at least three times a day, if not more.

Combine all that and your body automatically starts to feel fresher and healthier. This will also have a drastic effect on your personality. With more confidence, you will be able to deal with the public and lead a happier life.

Let's be honest, we all have a few things on our priority list which we cannot compromise on. One of them is sharing those intimate moments with our partner, right? The bad part is the libido, the thing that makes this magic possible, starts to drop low as we approach the half-century mark. Once we cross that, the fall increases drastically, and we feel the lack of urge for intimacy and a lower sex drive.

When something as important and pleasurable as sex dies out, life takes a toll. Without it, both men and women grow grumpy, irritated and lose their charm. While women have to worry about the menopause issues, men get to deal with things like erectile dysfunction. In either case, it is the stuff of nightmares.

With the help of keto though, things can change and change for the better. With a selection of some fine ingredients, you can cook up some food that will top your body up with the energy, strength, and the libido that you need to get back in action. Add to that a few exercises, and you would be as fit as you were quite a few years younger. Relive the moments with your loved ones and rekindle the fire that seemingly went out for good.

## Strengthening the Bones

One of the biggest issues' men face when they cross the magical number of 50 is the rapidly deteriorating strength within their bones. While they may have been able to walk for miles without breaking a sweat, back in the day, they would now face an incredibly tough time climbing a set of stairs no more than two stories high. This is an alarming situation, and one that needs a solution ASAP!

Fortunately, the keto diet provides some relief to the people suffering from joint aches from osteoarthritis and weakened muscles. Through this diet, the necessary nutrients are released into the body which will then cause a sudden spike within the body, brimming it with energy to carry out tasks that would otherwise seem impossible to do at such an age.

Imagine the keto diet as spinach for Popeye. The minute he eats it, he's all muscles. I should also point out that this is just a reference and that keto does not provide you with such quick results.

### Keto Helps to Prevent Certain Cancers

Cancer, whatever the type, is one of the most horrific diseases in existence. Just the mere mention of the word and everyone will immediately be stunned.

Cancers take time to manifest and are usually caused by long prevailing, underlying causes. They do not appear randomly and require the right kind of environment to develop. However, once they appear, time is of the essence. Be late and it is curtains for good.

With the introduction of keto, which was initially introduced within children to control epilepsy, things looked promising. While keto does not prevent all cancers, it is mighty effective against some types of cancers. Some reports have shown significant revival of patients who were aged 50 and above, which provides all the more reason for men above 50 to start on ketogenic diets, if they haven't already done so. Simply put, keto is possibly the only lifestyle men should seek to ensure a healthier life leading into retirement.

Some Side Effects You Should Know
Some of these side effects are universal, meaning that both men and women would face these. However, there are varying studies which suggest some symptoms or side-effects are more prominent within men above 50 as compared to women above 50. Nonetheless, it is a good idea to know what exactly you are dealing with and what you can expect to face as time goes by.

Most of these symptoms will fade away with time, but some may linger on. There is no such symptom that may pose a threat to you or anyone else. However, it is generally a good idea to be prepared to face these as they come. A prepared mind stands a better chance at dealing with things.

**The side-effects include:**

- The dreaded keto flu: A flu like illness that hits you right in the starting few weeks. Nothing to be alarmed about as this is only because your body is coping with the new changes.

- Keto breath: I do wish this was not the case, but since it exists, it is best to know of it beforehand. Keto breath is quite strong as it contains acetone.

- Tougher visits to the bathroom: You can either develop diarrhea or nasty constipation. However, rest assured, this is a short-term symptom and will go away shortly.

- A massive thirst: Yes! You will feel thirsty quite a lot. It is advisable that you drink plenty of water to ensure you do not suffer worse side-effects because of the added thirst.

As I mentioned, some of these symptoms may be more noticeable for men than women. However, the difference is marginal at best.

I had already warned the ladies to exercise caution before moving on and ensure that they check their conditions first and figure out if they have any special diet needs. Similarly, if men who are 50 and above face any issues, I recommend that you find out what you can eat and what you can't. You can consult a dietician or a doctor and get some details about what is good for you and what isn't. Once that is sorted, all you need is a pen and a notebook to start taking notes.

You will be spending a lot of time in the kitchen, so it is probably a good idea to hone in on your cooking skills. You will need them quite a lot if you truly wish to take benefits from the keto diet.

# Chapter 4: Keto for Women Vs. Men

In reality, since women and men have been created differently, our approach to Keto Diet may differ and should be different. These are the biological indifferences that we have no control with. We are going to be talking about the differences between males and females when it comes to approaching the Keto Diet.

So how should men do it or women do it? Here's a thing we need to understand about the Keto Diet first and foremost is that is very bio individual so that even among men, there are different ways to do it and among women there are different ways as well. So just understand that it is individual and it might take some tweaking as you go throughout the process. But for all men and for all women, it's really important to become Keto adaptive first before we start tweaking things so what we mean by that is you need to do Keto strict for the first thirty days or so until you get adapted. Your body is becoming more efficient and it is adapting to this new fuel source called ketones and it is going to take a while before your body gets adapted. But once you get adapted here is where there might be some difference in men versus women so some women tend not to do well over the long term with intermittent fasting.

So intermittent fasting is very popular that a lot of people that do Keto do intermittent fasting as well because it puts you in a modified or a modified state of Ketosis so you are making some ketones but women over the long term because of their hormones being different with men and their cycles during that time of the month. They might need to increase their carbohydrate intakes the week before their cycle starts.

So what we recommend to all women out there is that if you have become adapted to the Ketogenic Diet is that you should be cycling in and out of Ketosis from time to time and specifically try it out adding in healthy carbs, not talking about pizza, french fries or soda but healthy carbs like fruit, potatoes, sweet potatoes, maybe a little bit of rice the weak before your cycle. Adding thoes carbohydrates during night time could help out balance those hormones for you so that you don't experience there sideeffects from going Keto long term. And that is what we've seen help a lot of women that are clients is adding those in plus you are not as grumpy or angry. This stuff can definitely help out with those symptoms and side effects. So add in carbohydrates the week before your cycle.

For men also, it is best recommended that you test your hormones and get your blood work done every couple of months so you know how your body is changing and adapting so you know maybe you need to switch things up or maybe do the target aketogenic diet for a week or two and see how your body responds and adapts. You need to become your own experimentations so you know what is best for you moving forward.

The truth is, there is a wide variety of people who can benefit from the Ketogenic Diet, whether they are young, old, man, or woman, but the Ketogenic Diet has been known to be especially beneficial for women due to their different hormones and conditions. This diet can be especially beneficial for women who are:

- Lacking results on other diets

- Binge on carbohydrates

- Planning on getting pregnant

- Want a healthy pregnancy

- Struggling with irregular periods

- Struggling with sex hormones

- Going through menopause

When you first begin the Ketogenic Diet, you are most likely anticipating all of the benefits people mention. While those changes will come at some point, you should be aware of the dreaded Keto Flu. Unfortunately, many people do not anticipate for this metabolic change, and they are unable to push through the potential side effects.

With that in mind, you will want to remember that the Keto flu is only going to be temporary! The fly is most prevalent when the body is attempting to transition into the new, ketogenic state. As soon as your body learns how to be fat-adapted, the symptoms will disappear before you know it!

# Why Keto for 50+?

As we age, we naturally look for ways to hold onto our youth and energy. It's not uncommon to think about things that promote anti-aging. Products and lifestyle changes are advertised everywhere, and they are designed to catch your attention, as you grapple with the reality of what it means to be a 50+ year-old woman in our society. Even if you aren't eating for the purposes of anti-aging yet, you have likely thought about it in terms of the way you treat your skin and hair, for example. The great thing about the Keto diet is that it supports maximum health, from the inside out; working hard to make sure that you are in the best shape that you can be in.

For instance, indigestion becomes common as you age. This happens because the body is not able to break down certain foods as well as it used to. With all of the additives and fillers, we all become used to putting our bodies through discomfort in an attempt to digest regular meals. You are probably not even aware that you are doing this to your body, but upon trying a Keto diet, you will realize how your digestion will begin to change. You will no longer feel bloated or uncomfortable after you eat. If you notice this as a common feeling, you are likely not eating food that is nutritious enough to satisfy your needs and is only resulting in excess calories.

Keto fills you up in all of the ways that you need, allowing your body to truly digest and metabolize all of the nutrients. When you eat your meals, you should not feel the need to overeat in order to overcompensate for not having enough nutrients. Anything that takes stress off of any system in your body is going to become a form of anti-aging. You will quickly find this benefit once you start your Keto journey, as it is one of the first-reported changes that most participants notice. In addition to a healthier digestive system, you will also experience more regular bathroom usage, with little to none of the problems often associated with age.

While weight loss is one of the more common desires for most 50+ women who start a diet plan, the way that the weight is lost matters. If you have ever shed a lot of weight before, you have probably experienced the adverse effects of sagging or drooping skin that you were left to deal with. Keto actually rejuvenates the elasticity in your skin. This means that you will be able to lose weight and your skin will be able to catch up. Instead of having to do copious amounts of exercise to firm up your skin, it should already be becoming firmer each day that you are on the Keto diet. This is something that a lot of participants are pleasantly surprised to find out.

Women also commonly report a natural reduction in wrinkles, and healthier skin and hair growth, in general. Many women who start the diet report that they actually notice reverse effects in their aging process. While the skin becomes healthier and suppler, it also becomes firmer. Even if you aren't presently losing weight, you will still be able to appreciate the effects that Keto brings to your skin and face. Because your internal systems are becoming healthier by the day, this tends to show on the outside in a short amount of time. You will also begin to feel healthier. While it is possible to read about the experiences of others, there is nothing like feeling this for yourself when you begin Keto.

Everyone, especially women over 50, has day-to-day tasks that are draining and require certain amounts of energy to complete. Aging can, unfortunately, take away from your energy reserve, even if you get enough sleep at night. It limits the way that you have to live your life, and this can become a very frustrating realization. Most diet plans bring about a sluggish feeling that you are simply supposed to get used to, for example. But Keto does the exact opposite. When you change your eating habits to fit the Keto guidelines, you are going to be hit with a boost of energy. Since your body is truly getting everything that it needs nutritionally, it will repay you with a sustained energy supply.

Another common complaint for women over 50 is that, seemingly overnight, your blood sugar levels are going to be more sensitive than usual. While it is important that everyone keeps an eye on these levels, it is especially important for those who are in their 50s and beyond. High blood sugar can be an indication that diabetes is on the way, but Keto can become a preventative measure, that we've already talked about. Additionally, naturally regulating elevated blood sugar levels, also reduces systemic inflammation, which is also common for women over 50. By balancing the immune system, of which inflammation is a part of, common aches and pains are reduced. If, for example, you've noticed that you have been feeling stiff lately, even despite your efforts to exercise and stretching, this is likely due to a normal case of inflamed joints. Inflammation can also affect vital organs and is a precursor to cancer. Keto will support your path to an anti-inflammatory lifestyle.

Sugar is never great for us, but it turns out that sugar can become especially dangerous as we age. What is known as a "sugar sag" can occur when you get older because the excess sugar molecules will attach themselves to skin and protein in your body. This doesn't even necessarily happen because you are eating too much sugar. Average levels of sugar intake can also lead to this sagging as the sugar weakens the strength of your proteins that are supposed to hold you together. With sagging comes even more wrinkles and arterial stiffening.

If you have any anti-aging concerns, the Keto diet will likely be able to address your worries. It is a diet that works extremely hard while allowing you a fairly simple and direct guideline to follow in return. While your motivation is necessary in order to form a successful relationship with Keto, you won't need to worry about doing anything "wrong" or accidentally breaking from your diet. As long as you know how to give up your sugary foods and drinks while making sure that you are consuming the correct amount of carbs, you will be able to find your own success while on the diet.

As a woman over 50, you'll find that you will feel better, healthier and younger, by implementing the simple steps that will tune your body into processing excess fats for energy. You'll build muscle, lose fat, and look and feel younger. As we've touched on, a Keto diet helps balance your hormones, reversing and/or eliminating many common menopausal signs and symptoms.

# Chapter 5: What Is the Keto Flu?

As you probably could have already guessed, the Keto flu is fairly related to the regular flu. The Keto flu comes about because your metabolism is trying to adjust to running on your new form of energy, fat. This is going to be a drastic change for your body, especially because, for the majority of your life, it has been running off glucose or carbohydrates for energy!

When you begin reducing your carb intake, this is going to begin depleting the glucose stores in your body. This switch can be tough on your body, and from here, you will begin to experience the flu-like symptoms. If you have ever had the flu before, you already know that it is not a great feeling.

## Signs & Symptoms of the Keto Flu

So, what can you expect from this infamous Keto Flu? Some of the more common symptoms include:

- Low Energy Levels

- Sugar Cravings

- Lack of Focus

- Inability to Concentrate

- Irritability

- Heart Palpitations

- Insomnia

- Muscle Cramps

- Muscle Soreness

- Constipation

- Diarrhea

- Confusion

- Dizziness

- Nausea

- Stomach Pain

- Overall Brain Fog

If you are starting the Ketogenic Diet for the first time and are nervously awaiting the Keto-Flu, the symptoms listed above will generally start up around the first day or two of your diet. It should be noted that the length and strength of the symptoms are going to vary depending on the person. In fact, some people are lucky enough to skip the Keto flu altogether! Either way, you can rest assured that the symptoms will only last two weeks, at most. The sooner your body becomes fat-adapted, the better you will feel.

## Causes of the Keto Flu

As you expand your knowledge of the Ketogenic Diet, you should be aware that there are four main causes of the keto flu. We will go over each source in detail below to help you lessen the blow of the flu in the first place.

## Keto Adaption

Keto adaption is going to be one of the main culprits behind the Keto Flu. The body is incredibly complex and has two primary processes for energy. This includes glycolysis, which is burning glucose for energy and beta-oxidation, which is burning fat for energy. As your body adjusts, you will be switching from one process to the other. This switch is called your metabolic flexibility.

What many people don't realize is that genetics play a major role in our metabolic flexibility. If your metabolic flexibility is low, you are more likely to experience the symptoms of the keto flu. For this reason, some people handle the energy switch easier than others.

## Carbohydrate Withdrawal

When you first make the switch to the Ketogenic Diet, you can expect a number of symptoms like cravings for sugar, irritability, and mood swings. There are studies that suggest that our brain is affected by sugar, similar to the way that it is affected by drugs such as cocaine or heroin. When we eat sugar, it releases the "feel good," hormone, dopamine. If you are not getting your "fix," your body is going to protest.

For this reason, when you begin to reduce the number of carbs in your diet, you can expect some of these symptoms. If your diet is currently heavy in refined carbs, sugars, and processed foods, you may have it worse off than others. While this doesn't mean you should jump off the Keto wagon instantly, you should anticipate the flu before it happens.

Lack of Micronutrients

People who first begin the Ketogenic Diet may have a hard time finding the proper balance when it comes to their macronutrients and their micronutrients. I understand that it is difficult enough learning what you can and cannot eat, but these micronutrients are going to be important when it comes to your health.

As you begin the Ketogenic Diet, you already know that you are going to be cutting out a large number of grains, fruits, and vegetables. In order to make up for this, you will need to make sure you are eating a proper amount of keto-friendly foods that will still help you get your micronutrients in. Some of the best foods you can incorporate will be:

- Olive Oil

- Coconut Butter

- Fatty-cut Meat

- Seeds

- Nuts

- Fish

- Asparagus

- Spinach

- Eggplant

- Full-fat dairy

If you find yourself unable to get your micronutrients in, you may want to consider a supplement. Whether it is a multivitamin or a micronutrient powder, you will want to make sure that the item is free from additives, fillers, and sugars. This way, you won't have to worry about non-keto ingredients kicking you out of ketosis.

**Electrolyte Imbalance**

Last, but definitely not least, we have the electrolyte imbalance. When you begin to make the change of decreasing the number of high carb foods in your diet, you can expect your body to begin losing water at an extremely fast pace.

This happens because the glucose that is stored in your body is bound to anywhere from 2-3 grams of water. As your body begins to adapt, your cells are going to use up the stored glycogen, meaning that the water weight you have been holding onto is going to get flushed out.

When all of this water is flushed out of your system, it is easy to become dehydrated and suffer from an imbalance of electrolytes. Once you become dehydrated, you may experience normal symptoms such as fatigue, headaches, and muscle pain. You will continue to feel this way until you balance your system out again.

For this reason, it will be vital that you are replacing the water and minerals that you are losing during this adaption period. The important minerals you will want to consider include potassium, magnesium, and sodium. By increasing your intake of these minerals, it can help ease your transition period.

The good news is that you will not feel like this forever! These symptoms are only temporary and will reduce as you learn how to put your body into ketosis properly. The even better news is that you can help get rid of the keto flu faster than you thought! Below, you will find some of my favorite tips and tricks of getting rid of the keto flu and jumping into the benefits of the Ketogenic Diet.

## How to Get Over the Keto Flu

The anticipation of getting the keto flu can seem overwhelming, but the good news is that you are going to be able to help yourself. The reason people suffer from the keto flu for so long is that they have no idea what is happening to their body! Most people assume that they have to deal with the bad symptoms to get to the benefits of the diet. The truth is, these signs and symptoms from your body are like a cry for help! You don't just feel like junk for no reason! You will want to take the time to listen to your body and see how you can help yourself.

With that in mind, there are several steps you can take to help get you through the keto flu. Below, you will find some of my best tips to help you get over the keto flu and into ketosis with as little misery as possible.

## Drink Up and Stay Hydrated

The number one tip I can give you as you begin the ketogenic diet is to stay hydrated! Even if you think that you are drinking enough water, you probably aren't. Staying hydrated should be your top priority as you begin the transition period into ketosis.

As mentioned, water loss is to be expected as you begin your new diet, so these liquids need to be replenished simultaneously. The more often you are drinking, the easier the transition will come. You will see how much drinking water is going to reduce those awful symptoms of nausea, fatigue, and even those wicked headaches.

The best trick up my sleeve to help you drink more water through the day is to keep it in sight! I have a reusable water bottle that is by my side all day long. If you have a visual cue, it acts as an instant reminder to drink more water. I also suggest drinking a majority of the water during the day because it isn't so fun getting up to use the bathroom ten times a night.

## Think Electrolytes

While we are on the topic of getting enough water, you will want to keep in mind that balancing your electrolytes is going to be just as important.

Before the ketogenic diet, many people don't have to worry about their electrolytes unless they are highly athletic. As mentioned, your body is about to flush a mass majority of your water weight and electrolytes out of your system during this transition period.

With that in mind, it should be noted that people lose electrolytes differently. The good news is that there are several ways for you to mitigate this imbalance.

The first tip I have for you will be increasing your sodium intake! When you increase the sodium in your diet, this could help counterbalance the water loss that is happening in your body. With that in mind, you will want to consider a supplement of Himalayan pink salt rather than the table salt most people have in their house. You would be amazed at the additives found in simple table salt!

Next, you will want to consider eating keto-friendly foods that are rich in potassium. Potassium is in charge of energy production, body temperature, bladder control, heartbeat regulation, and even muscle cramping. If you find yourself having symptoms in any of these areas, you probably need to up your potassium levels. Some of the best sources of this will be pumpkin seeds, mushrooms, and delicious avocado!

Another mineral you will want to make sure you are getting is magnesium. When people have low magnesium levels, this could lead to insulin resistance and depression. To ensure you are getting enough of this micronutrient in your diet, you will want to include food sources like dark chocolate, macadamia nuts, pumpkin seeds, and salmon.

On the Ketogenic Diet, calcium is also going to be important. While most people think that calcium is only important for bone health, it is also vital for your cardiovascular health, muscle contractions, and blood clotting. For this reason, it is a good idea to consume calcium-rich foods like salmon, chia seeds, and leafy greens.

**Increase Fats**

When your body begins switching over to its new source of energy, you are going to want to make sure that you are providing it with enough fat! Unfortunately, many people are shy about their fat intake when they are first starting their diet because we have been told our whole life that fat is bad! Now that your body is no longer using carbohydrates and sugar as energy, you will need to give your body what it needs!

As you increase your fat consumption while reducing your carb consumption, this will help push your body into using the fat as energy. If you need, you can always supplement with MCT oil to help increase your ketone levels. It is also a good idea to up your fat source and includes foods such as:

- Coconut Oil

- Cacao Butter

- Olive Oil

- Heavy Cream

- Ghee

- Grass-fed Butter

- Avocado Oil

- Bacon Fat

- Walnuts

- Chia Seeds

- Pecans

- Flaxseed

- Fatty Fish

- Sesame Seeds

**Work it Out**

The next way to help get you over the keto flu will be exercise! This can be hard for some people, especially if they are unable to work through the symptoms provided by the keto flu in the first place. For this reason, I highly suggest light exercise anywhere from two to three times a week.

As you begin moving your body, this will help the switch drastically. As soon as you get over the keto flu, you will be able to resume your normal exercise routine. If you are first starting out, I highly suggest low-intensity exercises. You can try something like yoga, swimming, or even a light walk. With exercise, you will be able to boost your metabolic flexibility and get over the keto flu before you even know it.

# Preventing the Keto Flu

While it is beneficial knowing how to get over the keto flu, it is even better knowing how you can prevent it in the first place! If you are like everyone else in the world, you simply do not have the time to get sick! The good news is that there are some ways that you may be able to skip the keto flu altogether.

**Follow the Diet**

One of the main reasons beginners fall into the Keto-Flu is due to the fact that they are not following the diet the way they are supposed to! The keto diet best when you are getting the proper micronutrients as well as the right number of macronutrients.

The key to getting to your results is learning how to balance your nutritional needs. Yes, you could hit your macronutrients eating nothing but cottage cheese, but this is a sure way to dive right into the Keto flu. While it is going to be important for you to avoid carbohydrates, you will want to learn how to incorporate plenty of vegetables and seeds to help you get the nutrients you need.

**The Power of Sleep**

Unfortunately, many people are unaware of how important sleep is for the body. When you are first starting the Ketogenic diet, you will want to get at least seven to eight hours of sleep at night. When you are sleeping more, this could help reduce the fatigue and stress that comes along with the metabolism switch. If you struggle with sleep at night, you may want to consider a couple of power naps during the day!

Supplement

If you feel nothing is working, you can always consider taking a supplement or two. While, of course, you can get everything you need from a balanced diet, some people prefer the ease of a supplement.

# Chapter 6: Health Benefits of the Ketogenic Diet

As you can tell, there are some extremely complex biological processes behind the Ketogenic Diet. When you first start this diet out, you will want to consult with a doctor before you begin any changes. As far as any diet goes, it is crucial that you choose one that is going to benefit you rather than do more harm. For this reason, be sure to consult with a professional before you experiment on yourself.

With that in mind, why begin any diet if it isn't going to benefit you? Before you dive into the diet itself, let's learn all of the incredible ways that the Ketogenic Diet can help you. Whether you are looking to lose weight, gain energy, or improve brain function, the ketogenic diet may be just what you were searching for.

## Brain Benefits

As you begin to change the fuel source for your body, this includes significant fuel sources for your brain as well. Studies have found that through the Ketogenic Diet, individuals were able to increase the stability of their neurons as well as the up-regulation of the mitochondrial enzymes and brain mitochondria.

With that in mind, scientists have been studying how a Ketogenic Diet may be able to benefit those who have Alzheimer's disease.

It seems as though through diet, individuals have been able to enhance their memory as well as increase cognition. When this happens, a diet may be able to bring improvement to individuals with all different stages of dementia.

For those who do not need to worry about Parkinson's disease or Alzheimer's Disease, the Ketogenic Diet is also beneficial in increasing mental focus, clarity, and could potentially grant less frequent and less intense migraines. Generally, these conditions are related to altered brain chemistry and stable blood sugar levels, both helped by the Ketogenic Diet.

### Heart Disease

Another major benefit that makes people take a look at the Ketogenic Diet is the downstream effects of the diet on blood glucose levels. As you begin to cut carbohydrates from your diet, it can help keep your blood glucose stable and low. By doing this, individuals have been able to keep their blood pressure in check and are also able to lower their triglyceride levels.

When people first begin a Ketogenic Diet, they feel that it is counterintuitive to eat a higher percentage of fat in order to lower the triglycerides, but the truth is, fat has had a bad rep this whole time! In fact, it is eating excessive carbohydrates, especially fructose, that is the culprit behind increasing triglycerides! The truth is, through this new diet, you will be able to raise your good cholesterol and lower your bad cholesterol.

### Fight Cancer

When it comes to cancer, it is essential that you seek medical attention before you try to take your life into your own hands through diet. It is highly advised that you listen to your doctor's advice when it comes down to cancer treatment. However, there have been articles published based around cancer and the ketogenic diet.

In 2014, Dom D'Agostino's lab published an article based around ketones being able to decrease tumor cell viability in mice that had metastatic cancer. Within this article, it was found that, generally, cancer cells will express an abnormal metabolism that is characterized when glucose consumption is increased. When this happens, the genes begin to mutate, and the mitochondrial begins to malfunction. In the studies, it is found that cancer cells are unable to use ketone bodies as energy, therefore inhibiting the viability of the tumor cell in the first place!

### Improve Sleep and Energy Levels

Unfortunately, many individuals underestimate how important sleep is. The good news is that after only four or five days on the ketogenic diet, many individuals have reported that they already begin to benefit from higher energy levels. On a scientific level, this may be due to the fact that through your new ketogenic diet, you will be stabilizing your insulin levels. As your body becomes stabilized, this will help provide you with a ready source of energy rather than experiencing the spikes and crashes.

As far as sleeping goes, the ketogenic diet affects sleep are still being studied. Right now, it seems as though through diet, individuals are able to decrease the time they spend in REM and increase slow-wave sleep patterns. It is believed that this is due to a biochemical shift in the brain as your body learned to use ketones as energy. Either way, you will be sleeping more in-depth and longer than before, granting you a fresh start to each day!

## Decrease Inflammation

Inflammation is a strange defense mechanism used in the body to help the immune system recognize any damaged cells, pathogens, or irritants. Through inflammation, the body is able to identify these issues and begin the healing process. While this is beneficial for the most part, it, unfortunately, can persist longer than needed and will end up causing more harm than good.

If you have inflammation in your body, you may experience symptoms such as pain, redness, swelling, immobility, and sometimes even heat. But, these signs of inflammations only apply to the inflammations on the skin. Sometimes, inflammation can happen within our internal organs, and that is when we experience symptoms such as fever, abdominal pain, chest pain, mouth sores, and even fatigue.

Studies have found that the key player in inflammation, and the diseases associated with it, is suppressed BHB. Luckily through the ketogenic diet, BHB is one of the primary ketones you will be producing as you begin your new diet. This meaning that you will be able to help issues, including IBS, eczema, psoriasis, acne, and even arthritis, all through diet!

## Gastrointestinal and Gallbladder Health

If you suffer from heartburn or acid reflux on a daily basis, you may want to take a good, hard look at your diet. Unfortunately, many sugary foods, nightshade vegetables, and grain-based foods are major culprits of both heartburn and acid reflux. With that in mind, it shouldn't come as a surprise that when you change your diet to include low-carb foods, these symptoms will disappear almost instantly. The reason you experience these issues is through an autoimmune response, bacterial issue, and inflammation caused by these foods in the first place.

Another benefit of the Ketogenic Diet will be the altering of the microbiome found in your gut. An individual known as Dr. Eric Westman found that through diet, individuals are able to significantly reduce health issues as they change their microbiome. In fact, he believes that when you take away carbohydrates, this can fix just about any gastrointestinal issues that affect a number of different people.

Along those same lines, research has also found that carbohydrates may be a significant culprit behind gallstones as well. As far as the Ketogenic Diet goes, it appears that when individuals consume a diet that is higher in fat, this can help keep the system running smoothly and will prevent gallstones from forming in the first place.

Improved Kidney Function

Another common issue among the health community is kidney stones. The most common cause of both gout and kidney stones is due to elevated levels of phosphorus, oxalate, calcium, and uric acid in the body. Unfortunately, this is often combined with obesity, dehydration, bad genetics, sugar consumption, and alcohol consumption.

Through the Ketogenic diet, individuals are able to lower their uric acid levels and help improve the health of their kidneys. It should be noted that while the ketogenic diet can help long-term, this diet does temporarily raise the uric acid levels within the body, especially if you are dehydrated. While it does rise as the ketone levels rise, the uric acid levels will lower in about four to six weeks.

Improved Women's Health

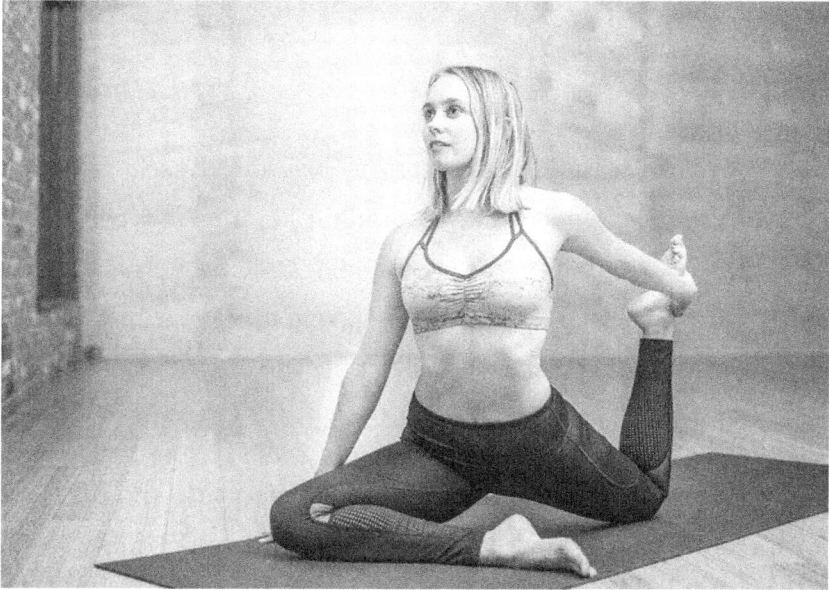

While the ketogenic diet is beneficial for both men and women, studies have shown that through diet, women may be able to stabilize their hormones and increase their fertility.

There was extensive research published in 2013 that looked at the key evidence linking ketogenic diets to enhancing fertility. It was also found that the Ketogenic Diet can treat PCOS (Polycystic Ovary Syndrome.) Through diet, individuals were able to eliminate or reduce symptoms of PCOS, including obesity, acne, and prolonged menstrual periods.

On a more general basis, it seems as though with this diet, individuals were able to keep their blood sugar levels low and stable. When this happens, it helps stabilize and equilibrate hormone levels, especially in women. Fortunately, this is a downstream benefit of the metabolic pathways that are related to insulin. Overall, individuals feel more balanced and stable than ever!

### Improved Endurance and Muscle Gain

As we get older, we generally begin to lose the muscle mass we once had. As mentioned, one of the main ketones you will begin producing as you begin the Ketogenic Diet is BHB. BHB is helpful in promoting muscle gain. When you combine the ketogenic diet with proper exercise, you will be increasing your health and muscle gain at the same time.

In addition to muscle gain, it is also believed that the diet can help improve endurance. Studies have found that athletes who switched to the diet and became fully fat-adapted showed significant improvements in both their mental and physical performances. Of course, this was compared to individuals who followed a typical diet that is rich in carbohydrates.

### Weight Loss

Weight loss is one of the major reasons anyone begins a diet. Luckily through the ketogenic diet, there is substantial evidence that by eating the proper foods, you will be able to lose weight and preserve your muscle mass. In a related study, it was found that individuals who followed a ketogenic diet, compared to individuals on a low-calorie and low-fat diet were able to lose 2.2 times more weight! In addition, these people also improved their HDL cholesterol and Triglyceride levels.

The best part about losing weight on the Ketogenic diet is the fact that individuals are still able to lose fat without restricting their calories nor controlling their food intake. This is important to keep in mind when it comes down to sticking to any diet. When individuals hate the extra work of counting their calories, they are statistically more likely to return to their old eating habits.

### Increased Metabolic Health

The last health benefit we will focus on increased metabolic health. Metabolic syndrome is described as give common risk factors for heart disease, type 2 diabetes, and obesity. These include high blood sugar levels, low levels of HDL "good" cholesterol, high levels of LDL "bad" cholesterol, abdominal obesity, and high blood pressure. The good news is that many of these risk factors can be eliminated or improved through better lifestyle and nutritional changes.

An important factor behind these issues is insulin. Insulin plays a vital role as far as metabolic disease and diabetes go. Luckily, the Ketogenic Diet is very effective when it comes to lowering insulin levels for individuals who are prediabetic or have type 2 diabetes.

In one study, it was found that after only two weeks following the

Ketogenic Diet, individuals were able to improve their insulin sensitivity by 75% and showed a blood sugar level drop from 7.5 mmol/l to a 6.2mmol/l! In another 16-week study, seven out of the 21 participants were able to stop their diabetic medication completely when they began the Ketogenic Diet.

As you can tell, the Ketogenic Diet can help a number of different people. While that is important to know, it is more important to understand how it works. The key to your success is going to be fat! While that may seem backward, what we are taught about fat is all backward! Yes, there are bad fats that we have to avoid, but good fat is going to be your new fuel source.

# Chapter 7: Keto Side Effects and How to Solve Them

It would be very irresponsible of me if I only tell you all the good things about the Ketogenic Diet and ignore the side effects. The truth is that there are negative effects that could happen once you start the Ketogenic Diet – but that's actually true for all of them! All types of diet have negative effects to start with because your body has gotten used to the bad habits. Once you make the shift to a more positive way of eating, the body sort of goes on a rebellious phase so it feels like everything is going wrong. For example, a person who used to eat lots of sugar in a day can have severe headaches once they start to avoid the sugar. This is a withdrawal symptom and tells you that your diet is actually making positive changes to the body – albeit it takes a little bit of pain on your part.

So what can one expect when they make that change towards a healthy Ketogenic Diet? Here are some of the things to expect and of course – how to troubleshoot these problems.

## Long Term Side Effects

A study titled "Metabolic Effects of the Very Low Carbohydrate Diets: Misunderstood Villains of Human Metabolism" shows that for short-term purposes, the Ketogenic Diet is very effective. It lets you burn all those excess fat quickly but in a healthy way. If you do this for a long period of time however, there will be side effects. For example, there can be muscle loss, dizziness, kidney problems, acidosis, and problems with focus. Does that mean you shouldn't go on a Ketogenic Diet at all? Of course not! This only means that you'll have to be careful when using this diet. Don't push it too hard and you will be able to get all the positive results with none of the downsides!

Do you know why a low carbohydrate diet is bad if done for a long time? Well, balance is important in anything you do and the Ketogenic Diet doesn't really support balance. If you get rid of an entire food group for a long period of time, your body will rebel against you. Remember – the Ketogenic Diet relies on stored fat in your body. If there are no more stored fat, it really won't work anymore so you will have to increase your carbohydrates. To solve this problem, I recommend going on a 30-day Ketogenic Diet first and assessing your health before moving forward. Asking your doctor what to do "next" after the 30-day plan or after hitting your weight goal is also a good idea. Personally, I decided to increase my carbohydrate intake slightly after hitting my goal weight.

## Keto Flu

The Keto Flu is the most prominent problem you'll encounter when starting the diet. It's a perfectly normal reaction by the body that may seem alarming because, well, the symptoms don't really feel good. You have to understand, your body has been running on a specific type of gasoline for years. It's been taking fuel from sugar and with the Ketogenic Diet, it's like you're changing your fuel source to a cleaner and more sustainable type.

It makes sense that the engine growls a little in protest – but after that, you'll be able to run beautifully without the guilt.

The Keto Flu has the following symptoms:

- Headaches

- Fatigue

- Irritability

- Brain fog or difficulty focusing

- Motivational problems

- Sugar cravings

- Dizziness

- Nausea

- Muscle cramps

- Frequent urination

These symptoms are all heavily dependent on the kind of person doing the Keto Diet. Since you're already in our 50s, the symptoms may be more prominent, especially if you rely heavily on carbohydrates in your diet. If you eat mostly low-carb food however, these effects may not be as obvious.

But how do you solve them? Here are some of the best way to get rid of the Keto Flu as quickly as possible!

First, increase your water and salt consumption. This happens a lot once you start a Ketogenic Diet. You may not notice it, but a lot of the salt you consume is through carbohydrates like bread, pasta, rice, and so on. Salt tends to make you thirsty so if you eat little salt, you're also less likely to look for water during the day. So what happens now? Every time you feel dizzy or tired or nauseous while on a Keto Diet, just dissolve salt in water and gulp it down. Now, this is not going to taste good - but I promise that it will help you feel better. You can always try consuming the salt and water separately – whatever you find most convenient. Beef stock, bone broth, or chicken stock are also great alternatives and tastier too! As for water, try to hit a target of 3 liters of water every day. The good news is that this doesn't have to be plain water – your smoothies, coffee, and tea drinks are also counted.

Add more fat in your diet. Because of all the wrong information circulating today, a lot of people are afraid of fat. Fat is not your enemy. During the Ketogenic Diet, it makes sense to eat lots of fats especially if your carbohydrate intake dips to an all-time low. If you lower the carbohydrate consumption without an equal fat increase, then you will always feel hungry and tired.

Don't be impatient – go slower. Remember what we said about the body changing fuels when you're switching to the Ketogenic Diet? Well, the changing process doesn't have to be overnight. Choose to convert one meal at a time to a Keto-friendly set instead of changing all of them on your first day. Of course, it's recommended that you only do this if the salt water method doesn't for you. Just remember – the Keto Flu will pass so the first few days of discomfort should not discourage you in the slightest. If you want to minimize the trouble, try starting your Ketogenic Diet on a low-stress period – like a holiday. So basically, instead of eating less than 50 grams of carbohydrates a day, you can have a target of 50 to 70.

Do NOT count calories or restrict your food consumption. When it comes to the Ketogenic Diet – you don't have to calorie count. Again, you don't want to just stuff yourself with food just because you don't have to count calories, but the truth is calories do not matter so much when your body is at a state of Ketosis. It doesn't matter so much how many you're getting – your body will always break down the fat deposits and there will be weight loss. Stressing about the calorie intake or depriving yourself of food because of the calories can actually worsen the symptoms of Keto Flu and will make it more difficult for you to stick to the diet. The bottom line is this: as long as you're eating the allowed food items in allowed portions, then you're OK.

Limit your physical activity. That's the good news with the Ketogenic Diet – you don't have to exercise. Sure, you may not be running marathons or going to the gym on a weekly basis, but if you're health-conscious, then chances are you do light walks on a routine basis. That's perfectly OK – as long as you don't over-exert yourself. Now, there will be days when you will actually feel too good. Like you can go out and exercise because you have all this extra energy. When this happens, resist the temptation to do too much too soon. Your body is already burning as much fat as it can – don't push it too hard or you might get sick. If you're restless, try doing yoga, light walking, or just stretching.

Take some supplements. People using the Ketogenic Diet for a long time may also have vitamin and mineral deficiency. It's not easily obvious but it could happen so you'll have to be prepared. The usual vitamins and minerals lacking in a Ketogenic Diet include calcium, zinc, selenium, and vitamin D – so try taking a multivitamin during your diet. Again, I can't stress this enough: always consult your doctor before taking any sort of medication. This is especially true if you have pre-existing health problems and are also taking medication for maintenance.

Constipation or Diarrhea

These problems are fairly common because, well, you're changing your diet! Your body will react one way or another and in both cases, the solution is practically the same – water and fiber. Make sure you get enough fluids in your system and take fiber supplements which is available through many stores. You can also try taking laxatives that are made especially without carbohydrates.

If alarming symptoms occurs while you're on the Ketogenic Diet, I want you to consult your doctor ASAP! Again, reactions may vary from one person to the next and I don't want you shrugging off certain symptoms as if they're just "part" of the diet. Stay motivated but also be mindful of what is happening to your body. Remember – we want you to be healthy!

# Chapter 8: Most Common Keto Diet Mistakes You Should Know

## The 9 Common Mistakes Beginners Do During Keto

Getting energy from fat, not sugar, is a very good approach and, as we have seen, can bring various health benefits. However, if you keep on the ketogenic diet every day, you can make some mistakes. If you know them, you can avoid them and realize their full potential.

### Give up before you stop ketosis

Food ketosis is a mandatory step and has more or less obvious and more or less long-term effects. They vary depending on how much carbohydrate has been abused before and how much our hearts are overloaded. When the body switches from burning sugar to burning fat, we feel like poisoned and weighed. They are poisons that rise and start blooming again after one or two weeks. Other symptoms associated with persistent ketosis include:

- halitosis

- a little nauseous

- early hunger for sugar

- fatigue

- nervousness

- a little sadness

These last symptoms are related to the effects of sugar and carbohydrate excretion on our mind, which makes us happy and satisfied by stimulating the same opiate receptors.

Conversely, if you stop them now and lose the allure, you might feel a little sad and nervous.

Many are afraid of these symptoms and are not well informed. They believe that the ketogenic diet is not for them, that they are worse off at the start and give up everything before they switch to ketosis.

## Lack of salt and minerals

The desire for sugar which was originally accused can be exacerbated by the possibility of mineral deficiencies. Therefore, they need to be integrated with the right dose of potassium, magnesium and sodium. Using Himalayan salt, eating salty snacks, using magnesium in the evening, could be just as many ways to remedy this mistake.

## Consume too much protein

At the beginning, higher doses of protein helps to overcome hunger crises, but then it is good to go back to consuming the right amount. To know how many proteins we should consume, just multiply our weight by 0.8 if we do normal physical effort and by 1.2 if we are sports. Another mistake regarding this category of food, which generally tends to be made, is that of consuming poor quality proteins, such as pork, cold cuts or putting different sources of protein on the same plate.

**Insufficient fat consumption**

This is another mistake that is easy to run into if we follow the ketogenic diet. We continue to be afraid of consuming fats and not using all natural sources: coconut oil, ghee, MCT oil, egg yolk, fatty fish, butter, avocado. The opposite mistake is to exaggerate with oilseeds: walnuts, almonds, flax seeds, pumpkin seeds that if we neglect to soak in advance with water and lemon, we also absorb the phytic acid they contain, a pro inflammatory substance and antinutrient.

**Consume bad quality food**

It is another of the most common mistakes. We focus on weight loss, but continue to consume frozen, canned, highly processed and, as mentioned, proteins that are practical and quick to eat, but of poor quality.

**Do not introduce the right amount of fiber**

Vegetables should always be fresh and consumed in twice the amount of protein and always cooked intelligently, that is, never subjected to overcooking or too high temperatures. In everyday life, if present, however, we often resort to ready-made, frozen or packaged vegetables. Also with regard to fruit, we often resort to the very sugary one, we forget that there are many berries with a low glycemic index: berries, mulberries, goji berries, Inca berries, maqui.

## Eat raw vegetables

I know this may surprise you, but consuming large quantities of raw vegetables, centrifuged, cold smoothies, over time slow down digestion, cool it, undermine our ability to transform food and absorb nutrients. This exposes us over time to inevitable deficiencies: joint pain, teeth, nails and weak hair, anemia, fatigue, abnormal weight loss.

## Consume the highest protein load at dinner

This is a mistake that involuntarily we all commit. The work, the thousand commitments, lead us to stay out all day, to eat a frugal meal for lunch or even not to consume it at all. Here the dinner turns into the only moment of the day in which we find our family members, we have more time, we are more relaxed and we finally allow ourselves a real meal complete with vegetables, proteins, sometimes even carbohydrates and then fruit or dessert to finish. It escapes us that even the healthiest protein, the freshest or most organic food, weighs down the liver. During the night, this being busy helping digestion, it cannot perform the other precious task: to purify the blood, prepare hormones, energy for the next day.

## Not drinking enough

And above all don't drink hot water. You got it right, drinking hot water is another story entirely, a huge difference from drinking it even at room temperature. The benefits are many: greater digestibility and absorption, deep hydration of cells, brighter skin and hair, retention disappears, cellulite improves, kidneys are strengthened, digestion improves, heartburn subsides.

# Ketogenic Foods

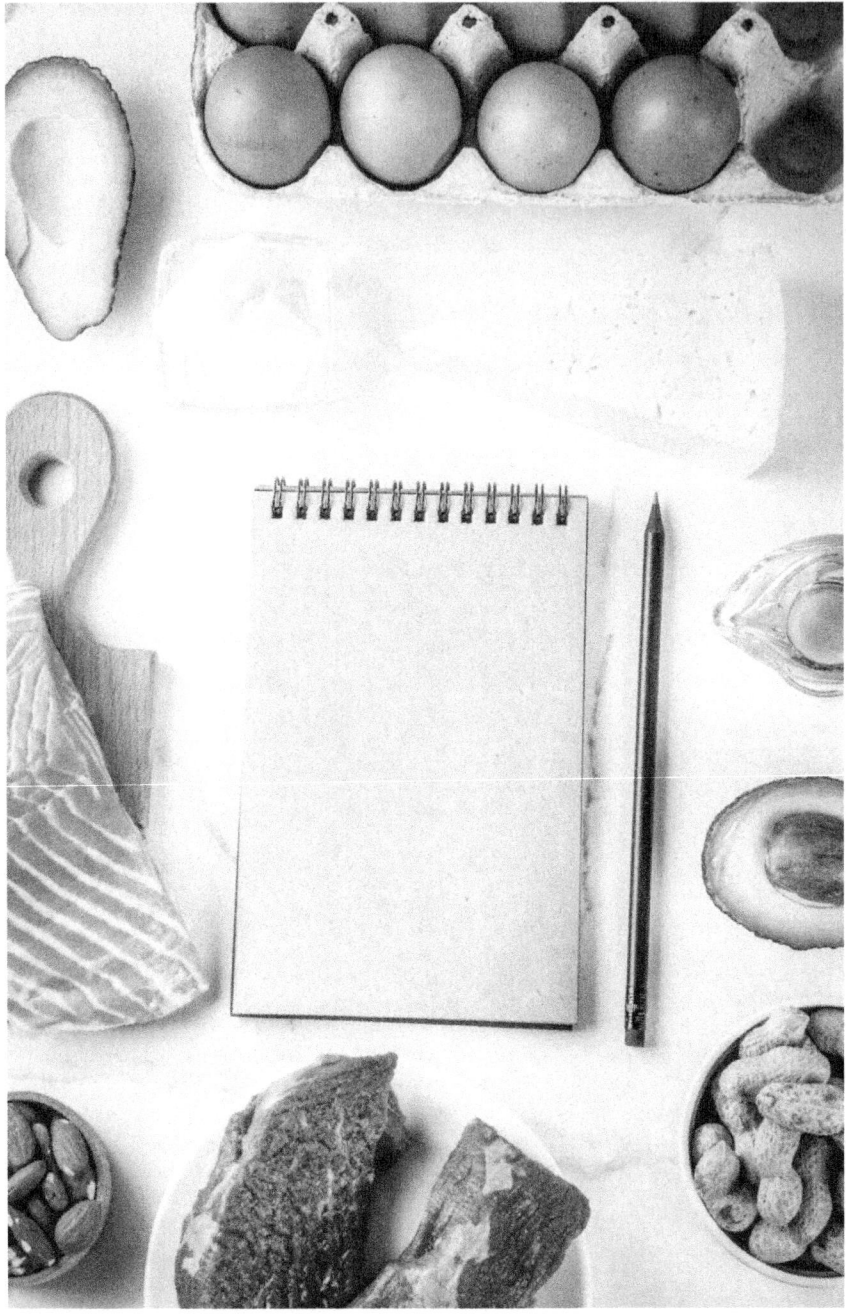

# Best Foods to Fit into the Keto Diet for Older Adults

I will go over what food you should consider incorporating into your keto diet. But the general guideline is that all foods that are nutritious and low in carbs are excellent options.

### Seafood

Fishes and shellfishes are perfect for keto diets. Many fishes are rich in B vitamins, potassium, as well as selenium. Salmon, sardines, mackerel, and other fatty fish also pack a lot of omega-3 fats that help in regulating insulin levels. These are so low in carbs that it is negligible.

Shellfishes are a different story because some contain very few carbs whereas others pack plenty. Shrimps and most crabs are okay but beware of other types of shellfish.

### Vegetables

Most vegetables pack a lot of nutrients that your body can greatly benefit from even though they are low in calories and carbs. Plus, some of them contain fiber, which helps with your bowel movement. Moreover, your body spends more energy breaking down and digesting food rich in fiber, so it helps with weight loss as well.

### Cheese

Milk is not okay. You can get away with cheese though. Cheese is delicious and nutritious. Thankfully, although there are hundreds of types of cheese out there, all of them are low in carbs and full of fat. Eating cheese may even help your muscles and slow down aging.

### Avocados

Avocados are so famous nowadays in the health community that people associate the word "health" to avocados. This is for a very good reason because avocados are very healthy. They pack lots of vitamins and minerals such as potassium. Moreover, avocados are shown to help the body go into ketosis faster.

### Meat and Poultry

These two are the staple food in most keto diets. Most of the keto meals revolve around using these two ingredients. This is because they contain no carbs and pack plenty of vitamins and minerals. Moreover, they are a great source of protein.

### Eggs

Eggs form the bulk of most food you will eat in a keto diet because they are the healthiest and most versatile food item of them all. Even a large egg contains so little carbs but packs plenty of protein, making it a perfect option for a keto diet.

Moreover, eggs are shown to have an appetite suppression effect, making you feel full for longer as well as regulating blood sugar levels. This leads to lower calorie intake for about a day. Just make sure to eat the entire egg because the nutrients are in the yolk.

## Coconut Oil

Coconut oil and other coconut-related products such as coconut milk and coconut powder are perfect for a keto diet. Coconut oil, especially, contain MCTs that are converted into ketones by the liver to be used as an immediate source of energy.

## Plain Greek Yogurt and Cottage Cheese

These two food items are rich in protein and a small number of carbs, small enough that you can safely include them into your keto diet. They also help suppress your appetite by making you feel full for longer and they can be eaten alone and are still delicious.

## Olive Oil

Olive oil is very beneficial for your heart because it contains oleic acid that helps decrease heart disease risk factors. Extra-virgin olive oil is also rich in antioxidants. The best thing is that olive oil can be used as a main source of fat and it has no carbs. The same goes for olive.

## Nuts and Seeds

These are also low in carbs but rich in fat. They are also healthy and have a lot of nutrients and fiber. They help reduce heart disease, cancer, depression, and other risks of diseases. The fiber in these also help make you feel full for longer, so you would consume fewer calories and your body would spend more calories digesting them.

### Berries

Many fruits pack too many carbs that make them unsuitable in a keto diet, but not berries. They are low in carbs and high in fiber. Some of the best berries to include in your diet are blackberries, blueberries, raspberries, and strawberries.

### Butter and Cream

These two food items pack plenty of fat and a very small amount of carbs, making them a good option to include in your keto diet.

### Shirataki Noodles

If you love noodles and pasta but don't want to give up on them, then shirataki noodles are the perfect alternative. They are rich in water content and pack a lot of fiber, so that means low carbs and calories and hunger suppression.

### Unsweetened Coffee and Tea

These two drinks are carb-free, so long as you don't add sugar, milk, or any other sweeteners. Both contain caffeine that improves your metabolism and suppresses your appetite. A word of warning to those who love light coffee and tea lattes, though. They are made with non-fat milk and contain a lot of carbs.

### Dark Chocolate and Cocoa Powder

These two food items are delicious and contain antioxidants. Dark chocolate is associated with the reduction of heart disease risk by lowering the blood pressure. Just make sure

they decide to take their own diet.

As always, those with health problems should consult their health care provider to help patients adjust to the meal plan or monitor them to ensure that their health is not affected by ketogenic therapy.

Keto diet is a low-carbohydrate high-fat diet with adequate protein in the meal. It is further broken down into three types, and depending on your daily calorie needs, the percentage varies. Diets are often prepared in a 4:1 or 2:1 ratio, with the first number showing the total amount of fat in the diet as compared to the combined protein and carbohydrate in each meal.

# Standard-SKD

The first diet is the Standard or SKD and is designed for people who are not active or who lead a lifestyle that is sedentary. The meal plan limits the dieter to eat a carbohydrate net of 20-50 grams. Starchy fruits or vegetables are limited from the diet. To be effective in the diet, the meal plan must be strictly followed. Butter, vegetable oil, and heavy creams are heavily used in the diet to substitute carbohydrates.

# Targeted-TKD

The TKD is less stringent than the SKD and allows you to consume carbohydrates but only in a certain portion or quantity that will not affect the ketosis you are currently in. The diet of TKD helps dieters performing some exercise or workout level.

# Cyclical-CKD

The CKD is preferable for those undergoing weight training or intensive exercises and not for beginners as it requires the person undergoing the diet to adhere to a five-day SKD meal plan in a week's time and to eat / load carbohydrate over the next two days. It is important for dieters to follow the strict regime to ensure a successful diet.

These are just a brief overview of the keto diet and would hopefully help you decide if you are interested in the diet. It is best to consult your health care provider for an in-depth discussion of the benefits and effects of the diet plan.

# Chapter 9: Fitness and Exercise: How to Lose Weight and Alleviate the Symptoms of Menopause

The first aspect that we have seen so far is nutrition. We say that a woman tends to consume less. The first thing we have to do is reduce the kcal that we have introduced. We try to keep a food diary for a week, we record each meal and relative grams, so we include everything in a nutritional application and try to reduce kcal by 5-10% next week.

Let's look at how it works and if the weight doesn't move, we reduce it by another 5-10% so we can reach the desired weight. We come to the second aspect, which is related to training. In this case, women must avoid all activities that can inflame.

Therefore, we avoid many repetitions, but limit ourselves to working with 3 series for each muscle group, 8 to 15 repetitions coming to feel muscle fatigue at the end of each series. This work will enable us to increase muscle tone without inflaming ourselves locally and systemically. Our advice is to exercise at least 2-3 times a week for 45-60 minutes to lose weight during menopause. The first thing you need to know: You need to determine what your goals are. This point is very basic: each physical activity has different characteristics and allows you to achieve different results.

Gymnastic activities with little consideration often produce results and tasks without stopping. So what are the main goals you need to have in your physical activity plan? I would say at least 3:

- help you burn more calories, keeping the cardiovascular system in shape

- help you strengthen the tissues that weaken most, i.e. MUSCLE and BONE

- help you prevent or solve problems typical of this phase, i.e. muscle pain, arthrosis.

Let's be clear right away: there is NO SINGLE activity that can make you achieve ALL these goals SIMULTANEOUSLY. You need a particular type of activity for each of these goals, and now I will explain just what type of activity. If for reasons of time or otherwise you will not be able to do everything, the world certainly does not fall, but at least you will know the reason why you do not reach a certain goal! In short, if you hoped that "an hour of walking + going to dance on Saturday evening" would have an invigorating effect for the muscles, prepare for a small (or big!) Disappointment.

One of the most desired and sought after goals through physical activity is that of slimming.

Losing weight is also one of the most "missed" objectives by the various users. The reason is simple: burning calories with physical activity is hard and time consuming, consuming too many with nutrition is very easy, painless and even pleasant. To help you with physical activity, you need something that allows you to burn a good number of calories.

Keep in mind that to lose fat, you need to take, on average, about 300 calories less per day than you consume. In an hour of walking at "medium" pace, you consume between 100 and 200 calories. And here is why, for most people, the famous "walks" do not have a significant impact on fat: to have a slimming effect, you should walk at least a couple of hours a day in a row. Walking is relaxing and is good for the cardiovascular system, but if your goal is to lose weight ... do your math well!

To get an idea, here is the "average" calorie consumption of various activities, calculated on an hour of activity and for a woman weighing 60 kg: if your weight is greater, keep in mind that consumption increases.

Remember: around 300 calories per day, so around 2000 calories per week. That's why "it's tough", and that's why you can't leave the diet behind.

- Aerobics course: 300 kcal / hour

- Medium speed exercise bike: 400 kcal / hour

- Travel at 8 km / h: 500 kcal / hour

- Swimming: around 500 kcal / hour

- Gardening: around 300 Kcal per hour

**Physical activity strengthens muscles and bones**

Other changes that women hate? There is clearly muscle loss, especially in the arms and legs. Can this muscle be restored? And how? And what can be done about osteoporosis? So, the answers to these questions are: yes, but it's not easy. And that looks. The reason is simple and to understand it, just focus on these two simple concepts:

- Muscles develop and tone only when asked about strengths

- Bones follow the same principle, that is, the more they strain, the stronger they become to tighten muscles and strengthen bones, you need activities that burden you.

Of course, they must be progressive and controlled overloads, but they are always overloads. Consequently, activities such as swimming, walking or cycling will not help you much: the overload (which is not fatigue, be careful!) To which the muscles are subjected is minimal. In fact, the only activity that allows you to strengthen muscles and strengthen bones is physical activity in the gym.

## Physical activity in the gym: recommendations

Physical activity in the gym should overload your muscles: Muscles will "register" and "adapt" to these new needs, will be strengthened. For this to happen, weighing a kilo and twisting with a stick are certainly not enough. Ask the trainer for a special muscle strengthening program.

## Physical activity to prevent or treat various problems

Menopausal women who don't have to deal with back or neck pain are counted on the fingers of one hand. Among other things, this problem often complicates physical activity: it is very difficult to lift weights when you suffer from back pain!

Therefore, part of your physical activity plan should aim to increase muscle and joint elasticity.

In this case, targeted stretches are extraordinary activities that you can do with other sports, among them. When you visit the gym, let your trainer show some exercise on important points, or contact a physiotherapist for professional advice. Conclusion: What physical activity should I choose?

If you follow my reasons, you understand one thing: one activity is not enough to reach all goals. And if you understand it correctly, it is not easy to achieve certain goals. It would be ideal to schedule activities throughout the day and throughout the week to cover all different aspects, but most people do not have time. So it's better to focus on what seems to be your main goal:

- do you want to lose fat? As you have seen, you have to grind kilometers!

- do you want to tone your muscles? Now you know that you have no alternative to the gym!

- do you want to solve the ailments first? Devote yourself to stretching and stretching, perhaps with the help of a professional

I understand that you may not like reading certain information: maybe you hate gyms, or you thought that walking half an hour in the evening could have positive effects on fat. Let's find out: Exercise is recommended, but certainly not an obligation! Now you know what physical activity is needed to achieve certain goals.

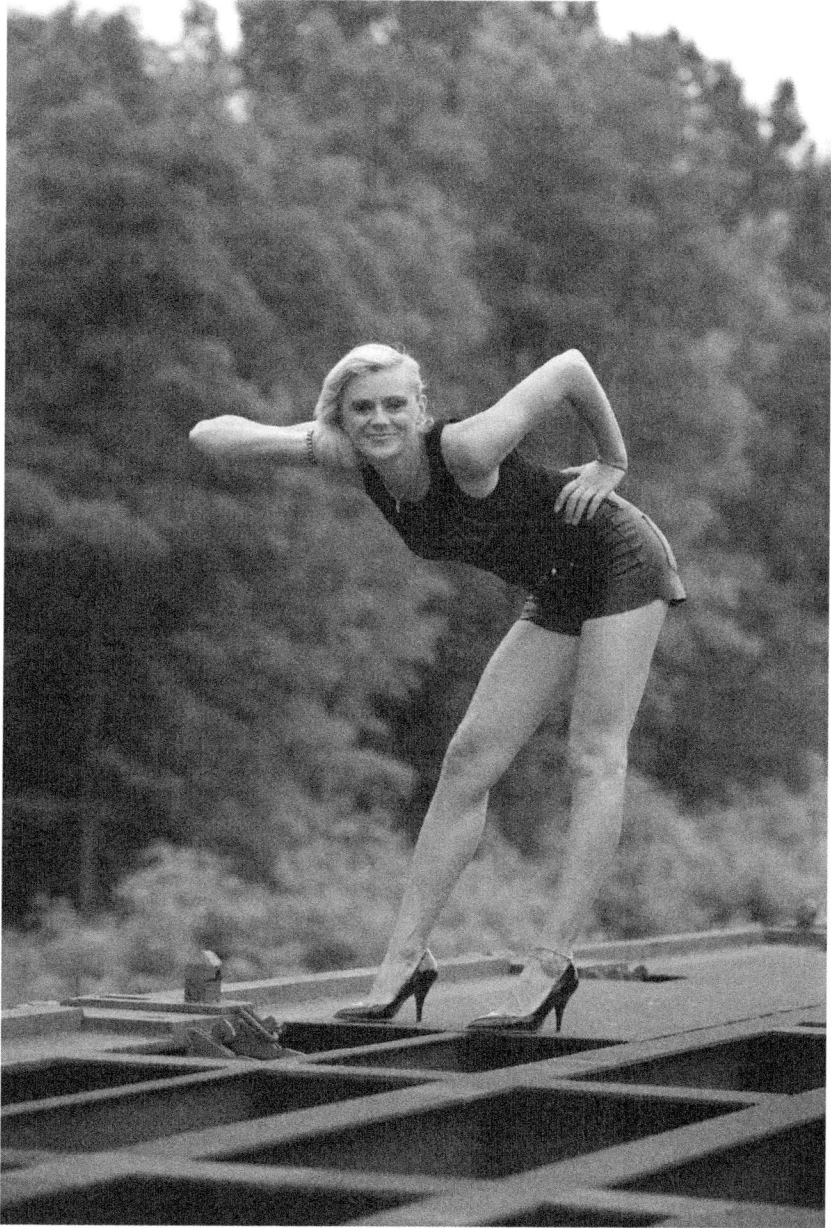

# Ketogenic Diet FAQs

## Why are you here?

OK – first things first – why are you here? I mean, why are you reading this book? Do you want to lose weight or do you want to just have a healthier lifestyle? This is an important question to ask and in all honesty, I feel like this is a question that we should have addressed in the first stage of the book.

If you'll notice, the book talks about how you can burn fat, lose weight, and prevent diseases with the Ketogenic Diet. Following this dietary plan will give you all three of these results – but finding out your ultimate goal will help you better plan your diet to achieve those goals. For example, if you're already happy with your weight and only want to have a healthier lifestyle, then you don't have to adhere so strictly to the carbohydrate requirement.

This is why I always encourage going to your primary physician first to find out what your dietary limits are. This was the first mistake I made when I decided to follow a weight loss regiment. Keep in mind – we're trying to improve the quality of your life and not make it worse.

## Is there such a thing as too much fat?

Everything in moderation. If you consume too much of one thing, it doesn't matter even if its water – it will be too bad for you. So yes, you can eat too much fat – even if it's healthy fat as already discussed. Remember how we talked about the importance of calories? Well, you have to understand that of all the nutrients found today, fat is perhaps the most compact type. This means that each gram of fat has more calories than any other nutrients you can find today.

What does this mean? This means that if you eat too much fat, there's a good chance that you'll go beyond your calorie requirements. If your goal is weight loss or maintaining a healthy weight, then this is a bad route to take because you won't be experiencing a calorie deficit. Simply put – you'd actually gain weight instead of losing it. I want you to understand this because I don't want you eating more than you should in the mistaken belief that its "healthy" for you.

**How much weight can you lose?**

The amount of weight you can lose on the Ketogenic Diet depends primarily on how well you stick to the plan. The healthy rate is 2 pounds per week and I strongly recommend that you don't speed it up too much. As mentioned, I lost 30 pounds on the diet – but this took years of hard work and personal research on my part!

**Should I be counting calories?**

Generally, counting calories is the go-to for people who want to lose weight. You will find however that this is not a problem when you're on a Keto Diet. That doesn't mean you should forget calories altogether – it only means that it's not that big of an issue in the grand scheme of things.

So the question is – how many calories should you be eating if you're on a Ketogenic Diet? Well, this depends from one person to the next. You will find that there are calculators that can help you get the proper amount of calories you want to maintain while on Keto. A good online calculator is known as the Mifflin St. Jeor calculator which allows for a calorie suggestion based on your height, weight, and age.

Of course, if you want to be challenged, here's the typical formula.

For males: 10 multiplied by weight in kilograms + 6.25 x height in centimeters less 5 multiplied by age + 5

For females: 10 multiplied by weight in kilograms + 6.25 x height in centimeters less 5 multiplied by age − 161

Once you get the results, you'll have to multiply it using the following situations:

- Sedentary: x 1.2, if you have minimal physical activities such as having a desk job

- Lightly active: x 1.375 light jogging at least once a week

- Moderately active: x 1.55 moderate activity, at least 6 times a week

- Very active: x 1.725 hard exercise daily or hard exercise twice a week

So it's a little tough − but the online calculator should make the whole thing easier. Generally however, you'd want to maintain a calorie count of 1500 calories per day for weight loss. For health maintenance without the need to lose weight, you can hit 1800 to 2000 calories – depending on the level of activity you experience every day.

Here's the most important question however: do you have to be strict about it? The short answer is: YES. Just because you're on the Ketogenic Diet doesn't mean you can eat all the meat you want. This is not a free pass – you still have to be mindful of what you eat.

The good news is that if you follow the Ketogenic Diet strictly, you'll find that the period of satiation is longer. Simply put, you won't feel hungry so quickly on the diet. There will be no mid-afternoon cravings for a snack as you feel full all through the hours between lunch and dinner. Even if you do feel hungry, there are a bunch of Keto-friendly snacks you can reach for.

## Primary Keto Guidelines – the Do's and Don'ts of Keto over 50

The Ketogenic Diet isn't as complicated as you would think. The general guidelines are simple and straightforward. Even for someone already in their 50s, the Keto Principle works just as well. Sure, there might be a need to make a few tweaks here and there to guarantee compatibility – but for the most part, everything one needs is easy to access.

What do we mean by that? Well, think about it – a person in their 50s is likely to have several maintenance medicines to help with their health. I know I've been taking several medications to help with problems like blood pressure, blood sugar, and so on. Once I made the decision to start a Ketogenic Diet, all of these medicines have to be taken into consideration. Like, is it OK to limit my food if I'm taking XXX medicine?

Of course, that's actually just one of the things I had to keep in mind. Here are other things you definitely have to consider when starting this brand new dietary lifestyle.

## Do Consult Your Doctor Beforehand

I can't stress this enough – especially for people who fall into a certain age group. Your general practitioner will know your medical history better, your current health status, and whether going on a Ketogenic Diet would be a good idea. It's important to remember that any diet has an impact on things like your mental health and psychological health. The change from a regular carb-full diet to a carb-free one can create pressure on yourself, not just physically and mentally. Simply put, this means that if you're under any sort of stress – the dietary change can do more harm than good. Your general doctor would be able to consider all these factors and give good guidance. At the very least, they can make slight changes to the Ketogenic Diet Principles to meet your health needs.

## Do Eat Less Than 50 Grams of Carbohydrates

The whole point of going on a Ketogenic Diet is to force the body to enter that state of Ketosis. To do that, one has to eat less than 50 grams of carbohydrates in a day. To put that in perspective, you should know that a single slice of white bread contains 49 grams of carbohydrates! Hence, people who are used to eating sandwiches for their meals are already eating way beyond the required limit. To let you better understand the low-carbohydrate principle, you should also note that the typical American eats around 225 to 325 grams of carbohydrates every day. For a healthy person with a normal weight, eating carbohydrates of around 225 to 325 is not a problem. For people trying to lose weight however, this amount should definitely be reduced.

**Do Increase Your Fat Intake**

When we say fat, we're talking about the healthy kind of fat. Try to stay away from products that are labeled as "fat free" because this is often packed with starchy ingredients.

**Do Eat the Good Kind of Meat**

Here's the good news for those following the Ketogenic Diet – meat is your friend. However, meat is you friendly only if it's the basic kind. What does this mean? Well, anything processed is not a good idea. You'd want to buy something that's as close to the real thing as possible. Sausages, hotdogs, and other meat products that went through a curing or preservation process are discouraged. If you can buy one directly from the farm, then that would be perfect.

**Do Avoid Excessive Exercise**

Especially during the first few weeks of keto, try not to exercise or do anything strenuous. I want you to focus on the diet to help yourself better stay faithful to the meal plan. This is because if you push yourself to exercise AND follow the Ketogenic Diet, there's a good chance that you'll fail in both. Pour all your willpower into keeping with the meal plans, even if you only do very little exercise during the week. You will find that even with this approach, you can still lose a significant amount of weight.

**The End Goal: Achieving Ketosis**

The end goal for the Ketogenic Diet is the same for everyone: achieving that state of Ketosis. That's the time when your body is getting energy from the stored fat instead of the readily-available sugar you eat on a daily basis – but you know about that already.

The real question here is – how do you know you're there? Because weight loss in the Ketogenic Diet may be quick, but it's not that quick! You will be able to observe other changes even before the weight loss begins.

# Chapter 10:     Keto Recipes

## Banana Waffles

Preparation Time: 30 minutes

Cooking Time: 30 minutes

Servings: 4 servings

Ingredient List:

4 eggs

1 ripe banana

¾ cup coconut milk

¾ cup almond flour

1 pinch of salt

1 tbsp. of ground psyllium husk powder

½ tsp. vanilla extract

1 tsp. baking powder

1 tsp. of ground cinnamon

Butter or coconut oil for frying

Directions:

Mash the banana thoroughly until you get a mashed potato consistency.

Add all the other ingredients in and whisk thoroughly to evenly distribute the dry and wet ingredients. You should be able to get a pancake-like consistency

Fry the waffles in a pan or use a waffle maker.

You can serve it with hazelnut spread and fresh berries. Enjoy!

Nutrition: each waffle contains 4g of carbohydrates, 13g fat, 5g protein, and 155 kcalories

# Keto Cinnamon Coffee

Preparation Time: 5 minutes

Cooking Time: 5 minutes

Servings: 1 serving

Ingredients:

2 tbsp. ground coffee

1/3 cup heavy whipping cream

1 tsp. ground cinnamon

2 cups water

Directions:

Start by mixing the cinnamon with the ground coffee.

Pour in hot water and do what you usually do when brewing.

Use a mixer or whisk to whip the cream 'til you get stiff peaks

Serve in a tall mug and put the whipped cream on the surface. Sprinkle with some cinnamon and enjoy.

Nutrition:

1gram net carbs

1gram fiber

14grams fat

1gram protein

136kcalories

# Keto Waffles and Blueberries

Preparation Time: 15 minutes

Cooking Time: 10 to 15 minutes

Servings: 8

Ingredients:

8 eggs

5 oz. melted butter

1 tsp. vanilla extract

2 tsp. baking powder

1/3 cup coconut flour

3 oz. butter (topping)

1 oz. fresh blueberries (topping)

Directions:

Start by mixing the butter and eggs first until you get a smooth batter. Put in the remaining ingredients except those that we'll be using as topping.

Heat your waffle iron to medium temperature and start pouring in the batter for cooking

In a separate bowl, mix the butter and blueberries using a hand mixer. Use this to top off your freshly cooked waffles

Nutrition:

3gnet carbs

5g fiber

56g fat

14g protein

575kcalories

## Baked Avocado Eggs

Preparation Time: 30 minutes

Cooking Time: 30minutes maximum

Servings: 4 servings

Ingredients:

2 avocados

4 eggs

½ cup bacon bits, around 55 grams

2 tbsp. fresh chives, chopped

1 sprig of chopped fresh basil, chopped

1 cherry tomato, quartered

Salt and pepper to taste

Shredded cheddar cheese

Directions:

Start by preheating the oven to 400 degrees Fahrenheit

Slice the avocado and remove the pits. Put them on a baking sheet and crack some eggs onto the center hole of the avocado. If it's too small, just scoop out more of the flesh to make room. Salt and pepper to taste.

Top with bacon bits and bake for 15 minutes.

Remove and sprinkle with herbs. Enjoy!

Nutrition:

271calories

21g of fat

7g fat

5g fiber

13g protein

7g carbohydrates

## Mushroom Omelet

Preparation Time: 15 minutes

Cooking Time: 5 minutes

Servings: 1 serving

Ingredients:

3 eggs, medium

1 oz. shredded cheese

1 oz. butter used for frying

¼ yellow onion, chopped

4 large sliced mushrooms

Your favorite vegetables, optional

Salt and pepper to taste

Directions:

Crack and whisk the eggs in a bowl. Add some salt and pepper to taste.

Melt the butter in a pan using low heat. Put in the mushroom and onion, cooking the two until you get that amazing smell.

Pour the egg mix into the pan and allow it to cook on medium heat.

Allow the bottom part to cook before sprinkling the cheese on top of the still-raw portion of the egg.

Carefully pry the edges of the omelet and fold it in half. Allow it to cook for a few more seconds before removing the pan from the heat and sliding it directly onto your plate.

Nutrition:

5 grams of carbohydrates

1 gram of fiber

44 grams of fat

26 grams of protein

520kcalories

## Chocolate Sea Salt Smoothie

Preparation Time: 15 minutes

Cooking Time: 5 minutes

Servings: 2 servings

Ingredients:

1 avocado (frozen or not)

2 cups almond milk

1tbsp tahini

¼ cup cocoa powder

1 scoop perfect Keto chocolate base

Directions:

Combine all the ingredients in a high speed blender and mix until you get a soft smoothie.

Add ice and enjoy!

Nutrition:

235 calories

20g fat

11.25 carbohydrates

8g fiber

5.5g protein

## Ingredient Zucchini Lasagna

Preparation Time: 20 minutes

Cooking Time: 1 hour 20 minutes

Servings: 9 servings

Ingredients:

3 cups raw macadamia nuts or soaked blanched almonds (for ricotta)

2 tbsp nutritional yeast (for ricotta)

2 tsp dried oregano (for ricotta)

1 tsp sea salt (for ricotta)

1/2 cup water or more as needed (for ricotta)

1/4 cup vegan parmesan cheese (for ricotta)

1/2 cup fresh basil, chopped (for ricotta)

1 medium lemon, juiced (for ricotta)

Black pepper to taste (for ricotta)

1 28-oz jar favorite marinara sauce

3 medium zucchini squash thinly sliced with a mandolin

Directions:

Preheat the oven to 375 degrees Fahrenheit

Put macadamia nuts to a food processor.

Add the remaining ingredients and continue to puree the mixture. You want to create a fine paste.

Taste and adjust the seasonings depending on your personal preferences.

Pour 1 cup of marinara sauce in a baking dish.

Start creating the lasagna layers using thinly sliced zucchini

Scoop small amounts of ricotta mixture on the zucchini and spread it into a thin layer. Continue the layering until you've run out of zucchini or space for it.

Sprinkle parmesan cheese on the topmost layer.

Cover the pan with foil and bake for 45 minutes.

Remove the foil and bake for 15 minutes more.

Allow it to cool for 15 minutes before serving. Serve immediately.

The lasagna will keep for 3 days in the fridge.

Nutrition:

338 calories

34g fat

10g carbohydrates

5g fiber

 4.7g protein

## Vegan Keto Scramble

Preparation Time: 15 minutes

Cooking Time: 10 to 15 minutes

Servings: 1 serving

Ingredient List:

14 oz. firm tofu

3 tbsp. avocado oil

2 tbsp. yellow onion, diced

1.5 tbsp. nutritional yeast

½ tsp. turmeric

½ tsp. garlic powder

½ tsp. salt

1 cup baby spinach

3 grape tomatoes

3 oz. vegan cheddar cheese

Directions:

Start by squeezing the water out of the tofu block using a clean cloth or a paper towel.

Grab a skillet and put it on medium heat. Sauté the chopped onion in a small amount of avocado oil until it starts to caramelize

Using a potato masher, crumble the tofu on the skillet. Do this thoroughly until the tofu looks a lot like scrambled eggs.

Drizzle some more of the avocado oil onto the mix together with the dry seasonings. Stir thoroughly and evenly distribute the flavor.

Cook under medium heat, occasionally stirring to avoid burning of the tofu. You'd want most of the liquid to evaporate until you get a nice chunk of scrambled tofu.

Fold the baby spinach, cheese, and diced tomato. Cook for a few more minutes until the cheese melted. Serve and enjoy!

Nutrition:

212 calories

17.5g of fat

4.74g of net carbohydrates

10g of protein

# Keto Snacks Recipes

## Parmesan Cheese Strips

Preparation Time: 30 minutes

Cooking Time: 30 minutes

Servings: 12 servings

Ingredients:

1 cup shredded parmesan cheese

1 tsp dried basil

Directions:

Preheat the oven to 350 degrees Fahrenheit. Prepare the baking sheet by lining it with parchment paper.

Form small piles of the parmesan cheese on the baking sheet. Flatten it out evenly and then sprinkle dried basil on top of the cheese.

Bake for 5 to 7 minutes or until you get a gold brown color with crispy edges. Take it out, serve, and enjoy!

Nutrition:

31 calories

2g fat

2g protein

# Peanut Butter Power Granola

Preparation Time: 30 minutes

Cooking Time: 40 minutes

Servings: 12 servings

Ingredient:

1 cup shredded coconut or almond flour

1 1/2 cups almonds

1 1/2 cups pecans

1/3 cup swerve sweetener

1/3 cup vanilla whey protein powder

1/3 cup peanut butter

1/4 cup sunflower seeds

1/4 cup butter

1/4 cup water

Directions:

Preheat the oven to 300 degrees Fahrenheit and prepare a baking sheet with parchment paper

Place the almonds and pecans in a food processor. Put them all in a large bowl and add the sunflower seeds, shredded coconut, vanilla, sweetener, and protein powder.

Melt the peanut butter and butter together in the microwave.

Mix the melted butter in the nut mixture and stir it thoroughly until the nuts are well-distributed.

Put in the water to create a lumpy mixture.

Scoop out small amounts of the mixture and place it on the baking sheet.

Bake for 30 minutes. Enjoy!

Nutrition:

338kcalories

30g fat

5g carbohydrates

9.6g protein

5g fiber

## Homemade Graham Crackers

Preparation Time: 15 minutes

Cooking Time: 1 hour 10 minutes

Servings: 10 servings

Ingredient List:

1 egg, large

2 cups almond flour

1/3 cup swerve brown

2 tsp cinnamon

1 tsp baking powder

2 tbsp melted butter

1 tsp vanilla extract

salt

Directions:

Preheat the oven to 300 degrees Fahrenheit

Grab a bowl and whisk the almond flour, cinnamon, sweetener, baking powder, and salt. Stir all the ingredients together.

Put in the egg, molasses, melted butter, and vanilla extract. Stir until you get a dough-like consistency.

Roll out the dough evenly, making sure that you don't go beyond ¼ of an inch thick. Cut the dough into the shapes you want for cooking. Transfer it on the baking tray

Bake for 20 to 30 minutes until it firms up. Let it cool for 30 minutes outside of the oven and then put them back in for another 30 minutes. Make sure that for the second time putting the biscuit, the temperature is not higher than 200 degrees Fahrenheit. This last step will make the biscuit crispy.

Nutrition:

156kcalories

13.35g fat

6.21g carbohydrates

5.21g protein

2.68g fiber

## Keto No Bake Cookies

Preparation Time: 15 minutes

Cooking Time: 10 minutes

Servings: 18 cook

Ingredient List:

2/3 cup of all natural peanut butter

1 cup of all natural shredded coconut, unsweetened

2 tbsp real butter

4 drops of vanilla lakanto

Instructions:

Melt the butter in the microwave.

Take it out and put in the peanut butter. Stir thoroughly.

Add the sweetener and coconut. Mix.

Spoon it onto a pan lined with parchment paper

Freeze for 10 minutes

Cut into preferred slices. Store in an airtight container in the fridge and enjoy whenever.

Nutrition: 80 calories

# Swiss Cheese Crunchy Nachos

Preparation Time: 30 minutes

Cooking Time: 20 minutes

Servings: 2 servings

Ingredient List:

½ cup shredded Swiss cheese

½ cup shredded cheddar cheese

1/8 cup cooked bacon pieces

Instructions:

Preheat the oven to 300 degrees Fahrenheit and prepare the baking sheet by lining it with parchment paper.

Start by spreading the Swiss cheese on the parchment. Sprinkle it with bacon and then top it off again with the cheese.

Bake until the cheese has melted. This should take around 10 minutes or less.

Allow the cheese to cool before cutting them into triangle strips.

Grab another baking sheet and place the triangle cheese strips on top. Broil them for 2 to 3 minutes so they'll get chunky.

Nutrition:

280 calories per serving

21.8 fat

18.6g protein

2.44g net carbohydrates

# Keto Dessert Recipes

## Keto Cheesecake with Blueberries

Preparation Time: 30 minutes

Cooking Time: 1 hour 30 minutes

Servings: 12 servings

Ingredient List:

1¼ cups almond flour (crust)

2 tbsp erythritol (crust)

½ tsp of vanilla extract (crust)

2 oz. butter (crust)

20 oz. cream cheese (filling)

2 eggs (filling)

1 egg yolk (filling)

½ cup of crème fraîche or heavy whipping cream (filling)

1 tsp lemon zest (filling)

½ tsp of vanilla extract (filling)

2 oz. fresh blueberries (optional)

Directions:

Preheat the oven to 350 degrees Fahrenheit. While waiting, prepare a springform pan by lining it with butter or putting in parchment paper.

Melt the butter until you smell that nutty scent. This will help create a toffee flavor for the crust.

Remove the pan from the heat and add almond flour, vanilla, and the sweetener. Mix the ingredients until you get a dough-like consistency.

Press it into the pan and bake for 8 minutes until you get a slightly golden crust. Set aside to cool.

Now we're going to work on the filling. Mix all the filling ingredients together and beat it heavily. Pour the mixture on the crust.

Increase the oven's heat to 400 degrees Fahrenheit and bake for the next 15 minutes

Once done, lower it to 230 degrees Fahrenheit and bake again for 45 to 60 minutes

Turn the heat off and leave it inside in the oven to cool.

Remove after it has cooled completely. You can store it in the fridge and served with fresh blueberries on top.

 Nutrition: each slice contains

4g net carbohydrates

 33g fat

7g protein

 335kcalories


## Keto Lemon Ice Cream

Preparation Time: 30 minutes

Cooking Time: 1 hour 30 minutes

Servings: 6 servings

Ingredients:

3 eggs

1 lemon, zest and juice

⅓ cup erythritol

1¾ cups heavy whipping cream

Directions:

Grate the lemon to get the zest and then squeeze out the juice. Set it aside in the meantime.

Separate the eggs. Using a hand mixer beat the eggs until they become stiff. Afterwards, beat the egg yolks and sweetener until it becomes light and fluffy.

Add the lemon juice in the egg yolks. Beat it before carefully folding the egg whites into the yolk.

In a separate bowl, whip the cream until you get soft peak. Gently fold the egg mix into the cream

Pour the whole thing into an ice cream maker and use it according to instructions of the manufacturer.

For those who don't have an ice cream maker, you can just put the bowl in the freezer. You'll have to take it out every 30 minutes to stir it. This should be done for the next two hours until you get the consistency you want.

Nutrition:

27g fat

5g protein

3g net carbohydrates

269kcalories

## Peanut Butter Balls

Preparation Time: 30 minutes

Cooking Time: 20 minutes

Servings: 18 servings

Ingredients:

1 cup of salted peanuts chopped finely (not peanut flour)

1 cup of peanut butter

1 cup of sweetener

8 oz of sugar free chocolate chips

Directions:

Mix the peanut butter, sweetener, and chopped peanuts together. You'll get a dough-light substance by doing this.

Knead until smooth and then divide the dough into 18 pieces. Shape them into balls.

Place the dough on a baking sheet lined with wax paper before putting them in the fridge to harden.

In the meantime, melt the chocolate chips in a microwave.

Take out the peanut butter balls and dip them in the melted chocolate. Put them back in the fridge to set. Enjoy!

Nutrition:

194kcalories

17g total fat

7g carbohydrates

1g sugar

7g protein.

## Keto Cake Donuts

Preparation Time: 30 minutes

Cooking Time: 30 minutes

Servings: 8 servings

Ingredient List:

6 eggs

½ cup coconut flour

¼ tsp sea salt

¼ tsp baking soda

1 tsp vanilla extract

¼ tsp almond extract

½ cup butter or coconut oil

½ cup erythritol

½ tsp of vanilla extract (frosting)

¼ cup melted butter or coconut oil (frosting)

¼ cup cream cheese, softened (frosting)

¼ cup powdered erythritol (frosting)

3 tbsp melted butter (chocolate drizzle)

2 tbsp powdered erythritol (chocolate drizzle)

1 tbsp cocoa powder, unsweetened (chocolate drizzle)

Directions:

Start by preheating the oven to 350 degrees Celsius Fahrenheit

Grab a large bowl and out in the donut ingredients.

Take a greased donut pan and will it with batter around 2/3 of the way

Bake for 20 minutes.

While waiting, start making the frosting. Do this by putting all the frosting ingredients in a bowl and stir completely with a hand mixer. Add sugar to taste.

Dip the now cool donuts in the frosting and set it on the parchment to cool.

For the chocolate drizzle, put all the ingredients in a small bowl and stir. Drizzle with the liquid as desired.

Nutrition:

294kcalories

2g net carbohydrates

4g fiber

28g fat

6g protein

## Chocolate Coconut Candies

Preparation Time: 30 minutes

Cooking Time: 20 minutes

Servings: 20 mini cups

Ingredients:

1/2 cup coconut butter

1/2 cup Kelapo coconut oil

1/2 cup unsweetened shredded coconut

3 tbsp powdered swerve sweetener powdered swerve sweeter

1 ½ oz. cocoa butter (topping)

1 oz. unsweetened chocolate (topping)

½ cup cocoa powder (topping)

1/4 cup powdered swerve sweetener (topping)

4 tsp vanilla extract (topping)

Directions:

Start by lining the mini muffin with paper liners.

Put the coconut oil and coconut butter in a saucepan and melt it using low heat. Stir completely before adding the shredded coconut and sweetener into the mix.

Divide the mixture onto the mini muffin cups. Set them aside so they'll become firm.

In a separate pan, put cocoa butter and unsweetened chocolate together. Melt them by setting the container in a pan of boiling water. This is done to avoid directly heat on the pan containing the chocolate.

Put the powdered sweetener and cocoa powder slowly until it smoothens into a thick consistency.

Remove it from the heat and put the vanilla extract. Blend carefully.

Spoon the chocolate topping on the firm coconut candies. Wait 15 to 20 minutes for it to set.

Nutrition:

240kcalories

5g carbohydrates

4g of fiber

25g fat

2g protein

6mg sodium

# Chicken Wings Black Pepper with Sesame Seeds

Preparation time: 8-10 minutes

Cooking time: 20 minutes

Servings: 2

Ingredients:

2 lbs. chicken wings

1½ tsps. salt

1½ tsps. black pepper

1¼ tbsps. ginger powder

1½ tbsps. minced garlic

1½ tbsps. extra virgin olive oil

½ tbsp. mayonnaise

1 tbsp. sesame seeds

Directions:

Place salt, black pepper, ginger powder, and minced garlic in a bowl then mix well.

Rub the chicken wings with the spice mixture then let them sit for about 5 minutes. Preheat an Air Fryer to 400°F (204°C).

Brush the chicken wings with extra virgin olive oil then arrange in the Air Fryer. Cook the chicken wings for 15 minutes then arrange on a serving dish.

Drizzle mayonnaise over the chicken wings then sprinkles sesame seeds on top.

Serve and enjoy warm.

Nutrition:

Calories: 207

Fat: 16.9g

Protein: 7.1g,

## Spicy Chicken Curry Samosa

Preparation time: 15 minutes

Cooking time: 30 minutes

Servings: 4

Ingredients:

1 lb. ground chicken

5 tbsps. extra virgin olive oil

¼ c. chopped onion

½ tsp. curry powder

¼ tsp. turmeric

¼ tsp. coriander

2 tsps. red chili flakes

2 tbsps. diced tomatoes

¾ c. almond flour

¼ c. water

Directions:

Place ground chicken, chopped onion, curry powder, turmeric, coriander, red chili flakes, and diced tomatoes in a bowl. Mix well.

Preheat an Air Fryer to 375°F (191°C) and spray a tbsp. of extra virgin olive in the Air Fryer.

Transfer the ground chicken mixture to the Air Fryer then cook for 10 minutes. Once the chicken is cooked through, transfer from the Air Fryer to a container. Let it cool.

Meanwhile, combine almond flour with 3 tbsp.s of olive oil and water then mix until becoming dough. Place the dough on a flat surface then roll until thin. Using a 3-inches circle mold cookies cut the thin dough.

Put 2 tbsp.s of chicken on circle dough then fold it. Repeat with the remaining dough and chicken. Preheat an Air Fryer to 400°F (204°C). Brush each chicken samosa with the remaining virgin olive oil then arrange in the Air Fryer.

Cook the chicken samosas for 10 minutes then remove from the Air Fryer. Arrange on a serving dish then serve with homemade tomato sauce or green cayenne.

Enjoy warm.

Nutrition:

Calories: 365

Fat: 30.3g

Protein: 23.1g

Carbs: 2.5g

# Garlic Chicken Balls

Preparation time: 8-10 minutes

Cooking time: 20 minutes

Servings: 4

Ingredients:

½ lb. boneless chicken thighs

½ c. chopped mushroom

1 tsp. minced garlic

1 tsp. pepper

½ tsp. salt

1¼ c. roasted pecans

1 tsp. extra virgin olive oil

Directions:

Cut the boneless chicken into cubes then place in a food processor.

Add roasted pecans to the food processor then season with minced garlic, pepper, and salt. Process until smooth. Cut the mushrooms into very small dices then add to the chicken mixture.

Using your hand mix the chicken with diced mushrooms then shape into small balls. Set aside.

Preheat an Air Fryer to 375°F (191°C).

Brush the balls with extra virgin olive oil then arrange the chicken balls in the Air Fryer. Cook the chicken balls for 18 minutes then arrange on a serving dish.

Serve and enjoy.

Nutrition:

Calories: 525

Fat: 46.8g

Protein: 23.7g Carbs: 5.7g

# Savory Chicken Fennel

Preparation time: 15 minutes

Cooking time: 40 minutes

Servings: 4

Ingredients:

1½ lbs. chicken thighs

2 tsps. fennel

1 c. chopped onion

¾ tbsp. coconut oil

1½ tsp. ginger

2½ tsp. minced garlic

1½ tsp. smoked paprika

1 tsp. curry

½ tsp. turmeric

½ tsp. salt

½ tsp. pepper

1½ c. coconut milk

Directions:

Place fennel, chopped onion, and smoked paprika in a bowl.

Season with salt, minced garlic, ginger, curry, pepper, and turmeric then pour coconut oil into the mixture. Mix well. Marinate the chicken thighs with the spice mixture then let them sit for 30 minutes.

After 30 minutes, preheat an Air Fryer to 375°F (191°C).

Transfer the chicken together with the spices to the Air Fryer then cook for 15 minutes. After that, pour coconut milk over the chicken then stir well. Cook the chicken again and set the time to 10 minutes.

Once it is done, arrange the chicken on a serving dish then pour the gravy over the chicken.

Enjoy!

Nutrition:

Calories: 414

Fat: 33.7g

Protein: 22.5g

Carbs: 6.4g

## Spicy Glazed Pork Loaf

Preparation time: 15 minutes

Cooking time: 30 minutes

Servings: 8

Ingredients:

1½ c. ground pork

½ c. diced pork rinds

½ tsp. paprika

½ tsp. pepper

2 tsps. minced garlic

½ c. chopped onion

½ tsp. cumin

½ tsp. cayenne

¼ c. butter

½ c. tomato puree

½ tsp. chili powder

2 tbsps. coconut aminos

½ tsp. Worcestershire sauce

1 tsp. lemon juice

Directions:

Combine ground pork and pork rinds in a bowl then season with paprika, pepper, minced garlic, cumin, cayenne, and chopped onion. Mix well.

Transfer the pork mixture to a silicone loaf pan then spread evenly. Set aside. Next, melt the butter in microwave then set aside.

Combine the melted butter with tomato puree, chili powder, coconut aminos, Worcestershire sauce, and lemon juice. Stir until incorporated.

Drizzle the glaze mixture over the pork loaf then set aside.

Preheat an Air Fryer to 350°F (177°C). Once the Air Fryer is preheated, place the silicon loaf pan on the Air Fryer's rack then cook for 20 minutes.

Remove from the Air Fryer then let it cool.

Cut the pork loaf into slices then serve.

Nutrition:

Calories: 255

Fat: 20.1g

Protein: 13g

Carbs: 6g

## Spicy Keto Chicken Wings

Preparation time: 20 minutes

Cooking time: 30 minutes

Servings: 4

Ingredients:

Chicken Wings - 2 Lbs.

Cajun Spice - 1 t.

Smoked Paprika - 2 t.

Turmeric - .50 t.

Salt - Dash

Baking Powder - 2 t.

Pepper - Dash

Directions:

When you first begin the Ketogenic Diet, you may find that you won't be eating the traditional foods that may have made up a majority of your diet in the past. While this is a good thing for your health, you may feel you are missing out! The good news is that there are delicious alternatives that aren't lacking in flavor! To start this recipe, you'll want to prep the stove to 400.

As this heats up, you will want to take some time to dry your chicken wings with a paper towel. This will help remove any excess moisture and get you some nice, crispy wings!

When you are all set, take out a mixing bowl and place all of the seasonings along with the baking powder. If you feel like it, you can adjust the seasoning levels however you would like. Once these are set, go ahead and throw the chicken wings in and coat evenly. If you have one, you'll want to place the wings on a wire rack that is placed over your baking tray. If not, you can just lay them across the baking sheet.

Now that your chicken wings are set, you are going to pop them into the stove for thirty minutes. By the end of this time, the tops of the wings should be crispy. If they are, take them out from the oven and flip them so that you can bake the other side. You will want to cook these for an additional thirty minutes.

Finally, take the tray from the oven and allow to cool slightly before serving up your spiced keto wings. For additional flavor, serve with any of your favorite, keto-friendly dipping sauce.

Nutrition:

Fats: 7g

Carbs: 1g

Proteins: 60g

# Cilantro and Lime Creamed Chicken

Preparation time: 10 minutes

Cooking time: 20 minutes

Servings: 4

Ingredients:

Chicken Breast - 4 Pieces

Red Pepper Flakes - 1 t.

Cilantro - 1 T.

Salt - Dash

Lime Juice - 2 T.

Chicken Broth - 1 C.

Onion - .25 C., Chopped

Olive Oil - 1 T.

Heavy Cream - .50 C.

Pepper - Dash

Directions:

If you are looking for a dish that is a bit different, this recipe is going to be perfect for you. Between the cilantro and the lime, this dish offers a fresh twist on traditional chicken. Many people feel that in order to lose weight, they need to give up flavor, but on the Ketogenic Diet, that is simply not the case! To begin this recipe, you will want to get out your cooking skillet and place it over a moderate temperature.

As the skillet heats, go ahead and season the chicken breast according to your taste. For this particular recipe, you will want to consider using the seasonings provided in the list above, but feel free to adjust levels to your own taste. Once seasoned to your liking, throw the chicken into the skillet and cook for about eight minutes on each side. When the chicken is cooked through, take it out of the pan and place to the side.

Next, you are going to add the onion into the hot pan and cook them for a minute before also adding in the cilantro, pepper flakes, lime juice, and the chicken broth. If you don't have chicken broth on hand, feel free to use water. Once these items are in place, bring to a boil for ten minutes.

Last-minute, you are going to whisk in your heavy cream and add in the chicken so that it can be coated in the sauce you just made. For extra flavor, add in some more cilantro, and then your chicken can be served by itself or with a keto-friendly vegetable!

Nutrition:

Fats: 20g

Carbs: 6g

Proteins: 30g

# Cheesy Ham Quiche

Preparation time: 10 minutes

Cooking time: 30 minutes

Servings: 6

Ingredients:

Eggs - 8

Zucchini - 1 C., Shredded

Heavy Cream - .50 C.

Ham - 1 C., Diced

Mustard - 1 t.

Salt - Dash

Directions:

Unlike traditional quiche, this version is crustless! Because there is no crust, this recipe offers a low-carb option for those who are still looking to make a savory meal for breakfast or lunch. For this recipe, you can start off by prepping your stove to 375 and getting out a pie plate for your quiche.

Next, it is time to prep the zucchini. First, you will want to go ahead and shred it into small pieces. Once this is complete, take a paper towel and gently squeeze out the excess moisture. This will help avoid a soggy quiche.

When the step from above is complete, you will want to place the zucchini into your pie plate along with the cooked ham pieces and your cheese. Once these items are in place, you will want to whisk the seasonings, cream, and eggs together before pouring it over the top.

Now that your quiche is set, you are going to pop the dish into your stove for about forty minutes. By the end of this time, the egg should be cooked through, and you will be able to insert a knife into the center and have it come out clean.

If the quiche is cooked to your liking, take the dish from the oven and allow it to chill slightly before slicing and serving.

Nutrition:

Fats: 25g

Carbs: 2g

Proteins: 20g

# Loaded Cauliflower Rice

Preparation time: 10 minutes

Cooking time: 20 minutes

Servings: 4

Ingredients:

Cauliflower - 1 Head

Cheddar Cheese - 1 C.

Bacon - 1 Lb.

Chives - .50 C.

Salt - Dash

Directions:

Sometimes, you just want something basic for lunch. This loaded cauliflower rice is fairly easy to make and only requires a handful of ingredients! The first step of this recipe is going to be ricing your cauliflower. You can choose to do this by hand, or you can purchase cauliflower rice in the frozen section.

Next, you will want to take several moments to cook your bacon. You can complete this task by heating a grilling pan over a moderate temperature and cook the bacon for four or five minutes on either side. I like my bacon crispy, but that is completely up to you!

When you are set, you are going to place your cauliflower rice into a microwave-safe bowl and sprinkle your shredded cheese over the top. When this is set, go ahead and pop the bowl into the microwave for a minute and allow for the rice to cook through and the cheese to melt.

Once the step from above is complete, top the dish off with your bacon pieces and season to your liking. Just like that, lunch will be ready for you!

Nutrition:

Fats: 10g

Carbs: 5g

Proteins: 5g

## Super Herbed Fish

Preparation time: 8-10 minutes

Cooking time: 6 minutes

Servings: 1

Ingredients:

1 tablespoon chopped basil

2 teaspoons lime zest

1 tablespoon lime juice

1 tablespoon olive oil

1 4-ounce fish fillet

1 rosemary sprig

1 thyme sprig

1 teaspoon Dijon mustard

¼ teaspoon garlic powder

Pinch of salt

Pinch of pepper

1 ½ cups water

Directions:

Season the fish with salt and paper. Arrange on a piece of parchment paper and sprinkle with zest.

Whisk together the oil, juice, and mustard in a mixing bowl and brush over. Top with the herbs.

Wrap the fish with the parchment paper. Wrap the wrapped fish in an aluminum foil.

Arrange Instant Pot over a dry platform in your kitchen. Open its top lid and switch it on.

In the pot, pour water. Arrange a trivet or steamer basket inside that came with Instant Pot. Now place/arrange the foil over the trivet/basket.

Close the lid to create a locked chamber; make sure that safety valve is in locking position.

Find and press "MANUAL" cooking function; timer to 5 minutes with default "HIGH" pressure mode.

Allow the pressure to build to cook the ingredients.

After cooking time is over press "CANCEL" setting. Find and press "QPR" cooking function. This setting is for quick release of inside pressure.

Slowly open the lid, take out the cooked recipe in serving plates or serving bowls, and enjoy the keto recipe.

Nutrition:

Calories - 246

Fat – 9g

Saturated Fat – 1g

Trans Fat – 0g

Carbohydrates – 1g

Fiber – 0.5g

Sodium – 86mg

Protein – 28g

## Beef Rib Steak with Parsley Lemon Butter

Preparation time: 8-10 minutes

Cooking time: 40 minutes

Servings: 4

Ingredients:

2 beef rib eye steak

2 tbsps. extra virgin olive oil

¼ tsp. salt

½ tsp. pepper

½ c. butter

¼ c. chopped fresh parsley

2 cloves garlic

¼ tsp. grated lemon zest

2 tbsps. lemon juice

1 tsp. basil

¼ tsp. cayenne

Directions:

Brush the beef rib eye steak with olive oil then sprinkle salt and pepper over the beef. Let it sit for about 30 minutes.

Meanwhile, place butter in a bowl then pours lemon juice over the butter.

Using a fork mix until the butter is smooth.

Grate the garlic then add to the butter.

Stir in chopped fresh parsley, grated lemon zest, basil, and cayenne to the butter then mix well. Store in the fridge.

Preheat an Air Fryer to 400°F (204°C) and put a rack in the Air Fryer.

Place the seasoned beef rib eye on the rack then set the time to 15 minutes. Cook the beef.

Once the beef rib eye is ready, remove from the Air Fryer then place on a serving dish.

Serve with the butter sauce. Enjoy right away!

Nutrition:

Calories: 432

Fat: 42.7g

Protein: 10.6g

Carbs: 4.1g

## Marinated Flank Steak with Beef Gravy

Preparation time: 8-10 minutes

Cooking time: 20 minutes

Servings: 2

Ingredients:

1 flank steak

¼ c. butter

3½ tbsps. Lemon juice

4 tbsps. Minced garlic

½ tsp. salt

½ tsp. pepper

1 c. chopped onion

¼ c. beef broth

2 tbsps. coconut milk

3 tbsps. coconut aminos

1 tsp. nutmeg

1 scoop Stevia

1 tbsp. extra virgin olive oil

Directions:

Allow the butter to melt in the microwave then let it cool.

Combine the melted butter with lemon juice, minced garlic, salt, and pepper then mix well.

Season the flank steak with the spice mixture then marinate for at least 3 hours. Store in the refrigerator to keep it fresh. Preheat a saucepan over medium heat then pour olive oil into the saucepan. Once the oil is hot, stir in chopped onion then sauté until translucent and aromatic. Pour beef broth into the saucepan then season with nutmeg. Bring to boil.

Once it is boiled, reduce the heat then add coconut milk, coconut aminos, and stevia tothe saucepan. Stir until dissolved. Get the sauce off heat then let it cool.

After 3 hours, remove the seasoned flank steak from the refrigerator then thaw at room temperature.

Preheat an Air Fryer to 400°F (204°C).

Once the Air Fryer is ready, place the seasoned flank steak in the

Air Fryer then set the time to 15 minutes. After 15 minutes, open the Air Fryer then drizzle the beef gravy over the flank steak. Cook the flank steak again and set the time to 5 minutes.

Remove the cooked flank steak from the Air Fryer then place on a serving dish. Drizzle the gravy on top then enjoy right away.

Nutrition:

Calories: 432

Fat: 42.7g

Protein: 10.6g

Carbs: 4.1g

# Buttery Beef Loin and Cheese Sauce

Preparation time: 8-10 minutes

Cooking time: 20 minutes

Servings: 3

Ingredients:

1 lb. beef loin

1 tbsp. butter

1 tbsp. minced garlic

½ tsp. salt

½ tsp. dried parsley

¼ tsp. thyme

½ c. sour cream

¾ c. cream cheese

2 tbsps. grated cheddar cheese

¼ tsp. pepper

¼ tsp. nutmeg

Directions:

Place butter in a microwave-safe bowl then melts the butter. Combine with minced garlic, salt, dried parsley, and thyme then mix well. Cut the beef loin into slices then brush with the butter mixture.

Preheat an Air Fryer to 400°F (204°C). Once the Air Fryer is ready, place the seasoned beef loin in the Air Fryer and set the time to 15 minutes. Cook the beef loin. Meanwhile, place cream cheese in a mixing bowl then using an electric mixer beat until smooth and fluffy. Add sour cream, and grated cheese then seasons with pepper and nutmeg. Beat again until fluffy then store in the fridge.

Once the beef loin is done, remove from the Air Fryer then place on a serving dish. Serve and enjoy with cheese sauce.

Nutrition:

Calories: 441

Fat: 39.4g

Protein: 15.7

Carbs: 5.6g

# Chapter 11: Meal Plan

A Keto Diet Meal Plan for women above 50+ years and Menu That Can change Your Body

The keto diet, generally speaking, is low in carbs, high in fat and moderate in protein.

When following a ketogenic diet, carbs are regularly diminished to under 50 grams for every day, however stricter and looser adaptations of the diet exist.

Fats supplies most of the carbs and convey roughly 75 percent of your all-out calorie consumption.

Proteins should symbolise about 20 percent of vitality, while carbohydrates are generally limited to 5 percent.

The decrease of carbohydrates forces your body to depend on its own energy which is fats for its primary vitality source to glucose — an event called as ketosis.

While in ketosis, your body makes use of ketones — particles delivered to the liver from the fat when glucose is minimized — as another fuel/enrgy source.

Despite the fact that fat is often maintained a strategic distance from for its unhealthy substance, explore shows that ketogenic diets are fundamentally more powerful at advancing weight loss than low-fat diets

In addition, keto diets decrease yearning and increment satiety, which can be especially useful when attempting to get in shape.

## Ketogenic Diet Meal Plan

Transferring to a keto diet can show to be overwhelming, yet it doesn't need to be that hard.

Your attention should be on minimizing carbohydrates while maximizing the fat and protein substance of meals and bites.

In order to be able to maintain ketosis, carbs must be minimized.

While some people may just accomplish ketosis by digesting under 20 grms of carbohydrates every day, some might be fruitful with a lot higher carbohydrates admission.

By and large, the lower your sugar admission, the simpler it is to reach and remain in ketosis.

This is the reason adhering to keto-accommodating nourishments and maintaining a strategic distance from things rich in carbs is the ideal approach to get thinner on a ketogenic diet effectively.

## Weekly Meal Plan

4 Week Meal Plan

| Days | Breakfast | Lunch/Dinner | Snacks |
|------|-----------|--------------|--------|
|      |           |              |        |

| 1 | Almond Coconut Egg Wraps | Cauliflower Mac & Cheese | Chocolate Avocado Ice Cream |
|---|---|---|---|
| 2 | Bacon & Avocado Omelet | Mushroom & Cauliflower Risotto | Mocha Mousse |
| 3 | Bacon & Cheese Frittata | Pita Pizza | Strawberry Rhubarb Custard |
| 4 | Bacon & Egg Breakfast Muffins | Skillet Cabbage Tacos | Creme Brulee |
| 5 | Bacon Hash | Taco Casserole | Pumpkin Pie Pudding |
| 6 | Bagels With Cheese | Creamy Chicken Salad | Chocolate Muffins |
| 7 | Baked Apples | Spicy Keto Chicken Wings | Lemon Fat Bombs |
| 8 | Baked Eggs In The Avocado | Cilantro and Lime Creamed Chicken | Vanilla Frozen Yogurt |

| 9 | Banana Pancakes | Cheesy Ham Quiche | Ice Cream |
|---|---|---|---|
| 10 | Breakfast Skillet | Loaded Cauliflower Rice | Chocolate Avocado Ice Cream |
| 11 | Brunch BLT Wrap | Super Herbed Fish | Mocha Mousse |
| 12 | Cheesy Bacon & Egg Cups | Turkey Avocado Chili | Strawberry Rhubarb Custard |
| 13 | Coconut Keto Porridge | Cheesy Tomato Shrimp | Creme Brulee |
| 14 | Cream Cheese Eggs | Cajun Rosemary Chicken | Pumpkin Pie Pudding |
| 15 | Creamy Basil Baked Sausage | Sriracha Tuna Kabobs | Chocolate Muffins |
| 16 | Almond Coconut Egg Wraps | Chicken Relleno Casserole | Lemon Fat Bombs |
| 17 | Bacon & Avocado | Steak Salad with Asian Spice | Vanilla Frozen Yogurt |

|    |                          |                                              |                              |
|----|--------------------------|----------------------------------------------|------------------------------|
|    | Omelet                   |                                              |                              |
| 18 | Bacon & Cheese Frittata  | Chicken Chow Mein Stir Fry                   | Ice Cream                    |
| 19 | Bacon & Egg Breakfast Muffins | Salmon with Bok-Choy                    | Chocolate Avocado Ice Cream  |
| 20 | Bacon Hash               | Buttery Garlic Steak                         | Mocha Mousse                 |
| 21 | Bagels With Cheese       | Baked Lemon Salmon                           | Strawberry Rhubarb Custard   |
| 22 | Baked Apples             | One Sheet Fajitas                            | Creme Brulee                 |
| 23 | Baked Eggs In The Avocado | Balsamic Chicken                            | Pumpkin Pie Pudding          |
| 24 | Banana Pancakes          | Cheesy Keto Meatballs                        | Chocolate Muffins            |
| 25 | Breakfast Skillet        | Beef Rib Steak with Parsley Lemon Butter     | Lemon Fat Bombs              |
| 26 | Brunch BLT               | Marinated Flank Steak with Beef              | Vanilla Frozen               |

|  | Wrap | Gravy | Yogurt |
|---|---|---|---|
| **27** | Cheesy Bacon & Egg Cups | Buttery Beef Loin and Cheese Sauce | Ice Cream |
| **28** | Coconut Keto Porridge | Chicken Wings Black Pepper with Sesame Seeds | Chocolate Avocado Ice Cream |

# Conclusion

Whether you have met your weight loss goals, your life changes, or you simply want to eat whatever you want again, here's the best way to come off the keto diet.

First, you need to prepare yourself mentally. You cannot just suddenly start consuming carbs again for it will shock your system. Have an idea of what you want to allow back into your consumption slowly. Be familiar with portion sizes and stick to that amount of carbs for the first few times you eat post-keto.

Start with non-processed carbs like whole grain, beans, and fruits. Start slow and see how your body responds before resolving to add carbs one meal at a time.

The things to watch out for when coming off keto are weight gain, bloating, more energy, and feeling hungry. The weight gain is nothing to freak out over; perhaps, you might not even gain any. It all depends on your diet, how your body processes carbs, and, of course, water weight. The length of your keto diet is a significant factor in how much weight you have lost, which is caused by the reduction of carbs. The bloating will occur because of the reintroduction of fibrous foods and your body getting used to digesting them again. The bloating van lasts for a few days to a few weeks. You will feel like you have more energy because carbs break down into glucose, which is the body's primary source of fuel. You may also notice better brain function and the ability to work out more.

.

# INTERMITTENT FASTING OVER 50

*THE STEP BY STEP GUIDE FOR BEGINNERS: THE 2020 ULTIMATE GUIDE WITH METHODS FOR SENIORS. RESET YOUR METABOLISM & WEIGHT LOSS.*

# Introduction

According to a study by Psychology Today Food and Wellness, 52 percent of Americans believe they find it much less complicated to learn taxes than to know how to eat healthy and balanced foods. Several people have difficulties with the current tax obligation code, which indicates that many more people have trouble discovering exactly how to consume a diet that is exceptional for them. We all understand that we should eat healthier foods. We are also aware that we must precisely limit the number of soft drinks, fruit juices, processed foods and sugars we consume, although we understand these things, this does not mean that it is so easy to follow. We live in a nation that has difficulties with weight problems. Two out of three adults are related as obese or overweight; the value that many people will surely fit into this ranking. Many elements increase weight problems. There has been a unanimous decrease in the quality of our dietary regimes as we move from a country that depends on regional agricultural food to a state where the mass produces most of our food. Since it is often conveniently offered today, this change has improved our food consumption.

Many easy-to-eat and straightforward foods are rich in fat, sugar, and calories. From the desserts, we discover in the bathroom to all the junk food chains that surround us, the quality of the food, and the amount we eat has changed significantly.

The problem with modern-day and fad diets is that it is simply not sustainable in the long-term. If you want to lose weight and feel better by yourself for the rest of your life, then you need to pick something which is not only sustainable but can be adjusted into your lifestyle based on your needs. Moreover, you need something that gives you the freedom to eat and have whatever it is that you like in moderation so that you can enjoy life and be with your friends and family a lot more often. The truth is, many fad diets do not allow you to eat food, which is unhealthy. Don't get me wrong; eating unhealthy food all the time is not the best thing for your body anyway.

Intermittent Fasting is a great option if you are desirous of burning body fat, lower weight, as well as developing better body shape. This diet plan is not only about the foods that you absorb. It is concerning the time of the day that you eat these foods to ensure that you can be well balanced and also healthy and balanced as well as additionally get your body to do the initiative for you.

An interesting thing to observe is that the intermittent fasting has a lot of supporters along with those who claim it is a useless technique. Why? For die-hard diet fans, the weight loss is not achieved without giving up certain foods. Intermittent fasting places zero restrictions on such diet restrictions, therefore, it doesn't seem effective to some people. However, that is not the case.

Most of the methods of intermittent fast revolve around limiting our meals and snacks to a specific time. The time frame is usually chosen between 8 to 6 hours within a day. In one of the methods, the meals are decided to be taken in any eight hours of a day while the remaining sixteen hours are to go without a food intake. Despite the claim of critics, the intermittent fasting has been proved by science. It provides many benefits including those of health, weight loss and general cholesterol.

So how does it work for weight loss? There are many mechanisms to prove that it does. Science has shown that the act of restricting your meals to a time window does wonders. The best wonder that it does is the reduction of calorie intake. It is a blessing for people who want to reduce their weight.

The calorie intake is quite important for weight loss. Usually, the weight gain is caused when calorie intake is more than calorie consumption. The extra calories are stored as fat. Thus, for weight loss, it is crucial that body functions are consuming the calories properly.

When the meals are restricted to a window of time, this restricts the intake of calories. It is a boost to calorie consumption. How? Suppose you do your breakfast. That will obviously lead to flow of calories in your body. When you plan your next meal within next eight hours, it will be another calorie intake. However, when you don't consume anything for the next sixteen hours, you are letting your body consume the calories that were taken in. Those calories are consumed properly and no extra calories are stored as fats. Your body will adjust to it more and more. It will naturally lead to weight loss. This is just one mechanism of how intermittent fasting works for the weight loss. There is also another advantage of intermittent fasting that actually ends up implementing weight loss effectively. That advantage is the increase in production of a hormone called, "neropinephrine". This is a special hormone that boosts metabolism. When your metabolism is faster, you end up digesting the calories effectively. This is a big boost to the weight loss. Furthermore, there is another benefit of intermittent fasting. It effectively reduces the hormone called insulin. This is often responsible for management of sugar levels in blood. The reduction of this hormone leads to more fat burning than usual. I don't think I need to link this to weight loss since it is quite obvious.

Furthermore, there is another benefit of intermittent fasting. That is the retention of muscle mass. Naturally when calories are consumed properly, not much is added to the fat ratio of body. This will lead to the retention of muscle mass that will naturally lead to better form. It is indirectly related to weight loss if your extra weight was caused by fat. There are many researches, which state that your body fat will reduce and weight loss will occur by intermittent fasting.

# Chapter 1: What is Intermittent Fasting?

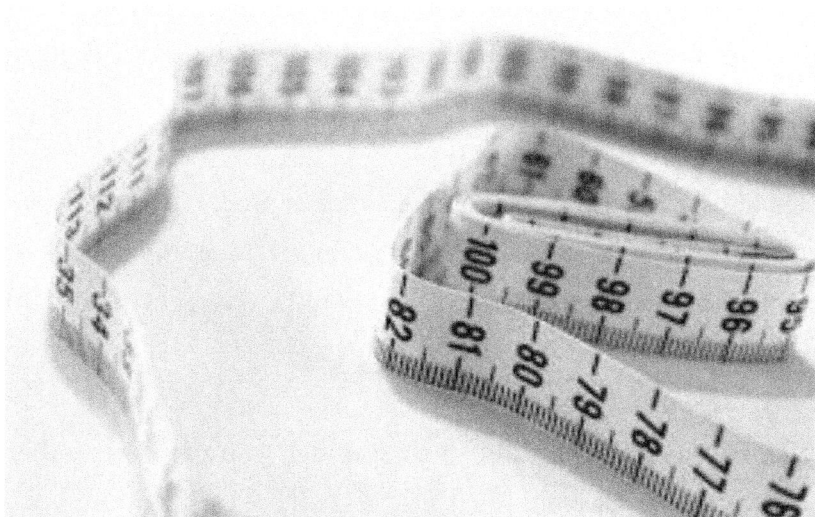

If we want to lose weight, we have so many diets that we often don't pay attention to how it works or what risks and benefits it has. One of the latest trends in the world of food is Intermittent fasting, which is very popular among athletes and is considered by many to be one of the most effective methods for weight loss. As the name suggests, intermittent fasting is a pattern that alternates between eating and fasting periods. Therefore, this is not the right diet, but a nutrition program that does not tell you what to eat and when.

There are a number of ordinary fasting methods and the most

popular are:

• Scheme 16/8: also known as the leangains method. This scheme divides the day into two parts: 8 hours of eating and 16 hours of fasting. It can be considered as an extension of the fast that is done automatically when you sleep, skipping breakfast and having your first meal at noon and then eating until 8.00 in the evening.

• On alternate days (5: 2): the idea of this model is that for two days a week the calorie intake is reduced to a maximum of 500/600 calories. The days do not have to be consecutive and on the other days you can eat whatever you want.

• Eat Stop Eat: according to this model, you eat every other day, once or twice a week.

On all models, you can drink low-calorie drinks such as coffee and tea without sugar.

**Why choose intermittent fasting?**
Experts have no doubts about the benefits of this practice: present in many cultures for centuries - abstinence from food helps the body attack excess fat: the cells, put in a stick, will go in search of the stored fat to be used as fuel, giving an incredible acceleration to the metabolism. After about 12 hours of fasting, the body will have exhausted the glucose present in the blood and that stored in the form of glycogen in the liver and muscles. Running out of energy, our body will be forced to burn fat to

meet all its needs.

Intermittent fasting has been a topic of discussion for lot of time. The first study is about reducing calories to strengthen body. Reducing energy supply is seen as a "hermetic" stimulus. A small amount of stress can increase cell endurance. Intermittent feeding contributes to the calorie factor, which prolongs fasting status, thus maintaining the status of certain hormones for a long time, with very low insulin levels. It seems that scientific evidence shows that this approach can effectively optimize metabolism while slowing down aging. It is also fair to say that further confirmation is needed.

With intermittent intervals eating, food intake is isolated for a certain period of time and hunger remains for the rest of the time, experts continue. In general, the so-called 16/8 regime is practiced, that is, 16 hours without food, with food concentrated on the remaining 8 hours. It's generally a matter of skipping dinner or breakfast, depending on your preferences.

It is important to remember that no form of abstinence from food can compensate for damage caused by poor nutrition. Therefore, even with intermittent fasting, it is important that the hours you eat are balanced and prefer vegetables, fruits, whole grains, nuts, fish, lean meats and healthy fats, like extra virgin olive oil. However, it is wrong to look for performance in the sugar, beverage, and food industries that endanger health and lines. The risk should not be underestimated, especially if you have lots of pounds to lose. However, nothing is excessive.

## Make Intermittent Fast to lose weight

Skipping meals creates a calorie deficit and hence weight loss. Of course, as long as you don't balance the fasting period with foods that are high in sugar or fat, because this type of diet doesn't say exactly what you can and can't eat. Studies show that regular fasting, when used correctly, also helps prevent type 2 diabetes and the body learns to process digested food more efficiently. Other studies also show that combination of strength training and the 16/8 method allows you to reduce your body fat percentage beyond what is eliminated by exercise alone. Therefore, it seems very effective when combined with regular exercise.

Note, important. This type of diet is not suitable for diabetics or high blood pressure, as well as for pregnant women or nursing mothers. It is best to consult with a doctor before practicing this type of diet.

Intermittent fasting can help you lose weight but if you are a woman with an active social life, you need to consider this so start this diet. If planned, the diet allows you to eat together with friends and relatives, but in general, it does not leave much room for flexibility and spontaneity. If the social aspect is important, it is better to follow a so-called Flexitarian diet (also known as a flexible diet or IIFYM).

Many women who follow this type of diet complain of hunger and fatigue, which can easily occur if they skip meals. But some say that after a critical phase, (about 2-3 days) hunger disappears. If you are too hungry, you can drink green tea or black coffee so you can hold yourself until the next meal. Regular fasting is not for everyone, but is a good way to reduce body fat. However, you need to control your diet and avoid burgers, pizza, and French fries. The goal is to keep eating healthy and eating a balanced diet.

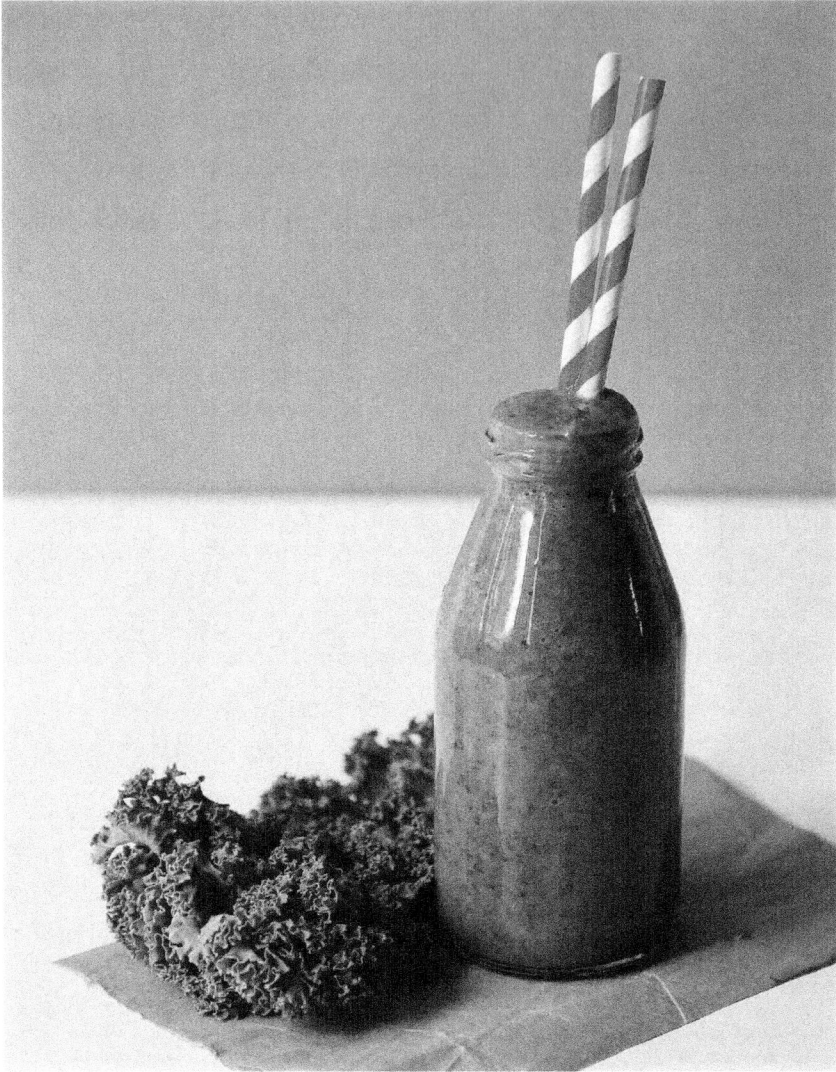

# Chapter 2: Different     Types     of Intermittent Fasting

## 16/8 Method

This is one of the most popular methods of fasting because it is so schedule based, meaning there are no surprises. This gives you the freedom to control when you eat based on your daily life. The 16 is the number of hours you are going to be fasting, which can also be lowered to 12 or 14 hours if that fits into your life better. Then your eating period will be between 8 and 10 hours each day. This might seem daunting, but it really just means that you are skipping an entire meal. Many people choose to begin their fast around 7 or 8 p.m. and then do not eat until 11 or noon the next day, which means they are fasting for the recommended 16 hours. Of course, it isn't as bad as it sounds since they are also sleeping during this time too, so what it really comes down to is eating dinner and then not eating again the next day around lunch, so you are just skipping breakfast.

You will be doing every day, so finding the hours that work for you are important. If you work third shift, then switching your eating period around to fit into your schedule is important. Also, if you find yourself being run down and sluggish, then tweak your fasting hours until you find a healthy balance. Granted, there is going to be some adjustment, because, chances are, your body is not accustomed to skipping entire meals. However, this should go away after a couple of weeks, and if it doesn't then try starting your fasting period earlier in the day allowing you to eat earlier the next, or alter it however you need to feel healthy and happy.

## Lean-Gains Method (14:10)

The lean-gains method has several different incarnations on the web, but its fame comes from the fact that it helps shed fat while building it into muscle almost immediately. Through the lean-gains method, you'll find yourself able to shift all that fat to be muscle through a rigorous practice of fasting, eating right, and exercising.

Through this method, you fast anywhere from 14 to 16 hours and then spend the remaining 10 or 8 hours each day engaged in eating and exercise. This method, as opposed to the crescendo, features daily fasting and eating, rather than alternated days of eating versus not. Therefore, you don't have to be quite so cautious about extending the physical effort to exercise on the days you are fasting because those days when you're fasting are literally every day!

For the lean-gains method, start fasting only 14 hours and work it up to 16 if you feel comfortable with it, but never forget to drink enough water and be careful about expending too much energy on exercise! Remember that you want to grow in health and potential through intermittent fasting. You'll certainly not want to lose any of that growth by forcing the process along.

## 20:4 Method

Stepping things up a notch from the 14:10 and 16:8 methods, the

20:4 method is a tough one to master, for it is rather unforgiving. People talk about this method of intermittent fasting as intense and highly restrictive, but they also say that the effects of living this method are almost unparalleled with all other tactics.

For the 20:4 method, you'll fast for 20 hours each day and squeeze all your meals, all your eating, and all your snacking into 4 hours. People who attempt 20:4 normally have two smaller meals or just one large meal and a few snacks during their 4-hour window to eat, and it really is up to the individual which four hours of the day they devote to eating.

The trick for this method is to make sure you're not overeating or bingeing during those 4-hour windows to eat. It is all-too-easy to get hungry during the 20-hour fast and have that feeling then propel you into intense and unrealistic hunger or meal sizes after the fast period is over. Be careful if you try this method. If you're new to intermittent fasting, work your way up to this one gradually, and if you're working your way up already, only make the shift to 20:4 when you know you're ready. It would surely disappoint if all your progress with intermittent fasting got hijacked by one poorly thought-out goal with 20:4 method.

## Meal Skipping

Meal skipping is an extremely flexible form of intermittent fasting that can provide all of the benefits of intermittent fasting but with less of the strict scheduling. If you are not someone who has a typical schedule or who feels as though a more strict variation of the intermittent fasting diet will serve you, meal skipping is a viable alternative.

Many people who choose to use meal skipping find it to be a great way to listen to their body and follow their basic instincts. If they are not hungry, they simply don't eat that meal. Instead, they wait for the next one. Meal skipping can also be helpful for people who have time constraints and who may not always be able to get in a certain meal of the day.

It is important to realize that with meal skipping, you may not always be maintaining a 10-16-hour window of fasting. As a result, you may not get every benefit that comes from other fasting diets. However, this may be a great solution to people who want an intermittent fasting diet that feels more natural to them. It may also be a great idea for those who are looking to begin listening to their body more so that they can adjust to a more intense variation of the diet with greater ease. In other words, it can be a great transitional diet for you if you are not ready to jump into one of the other fasting diets just yet.

## Warrior Diet Fasting

The most extreme form of intermittent fasting is known as the Warrior Diet. This intermittent fasting cycle follows a 20-hour fasting window with a short 4-hour eating window. During that eating window, individuals are supposed to only consume raw fruits and vegetables. They can also eat one large meal. Typically, the eating window takes place at night time so people can snack throughout the evening, have a large meal, and then resume fasting.

Because of the length of fasting taking place during the Warrior Diet, people should also consume a fairly hearty level of healthy fats. Doing so will give the body something to consume during the fast to produce energy with. A small amount of carbohydrates can also be incorporated to support energy levels, too.

People who eat the Warrior Diet tend to believe that humans are natural nocturnal eaters and that we are not meant to eat throughout the day. The belief is that eating this way follows our natural circadian rhythms, allowing our body to work optimally.

The only people who should consider doing the Warrior Diet are those who have already had success with other forms of intermittent fasting and who are used to it. Attempting to jump straight into the Warrior Diet can have serious repercussions for anyone who is not used to intermittent fasting. Even still, those who are used to it may find this particular style to be too extreme for them to maintain.

## Eat-Stop-Eat (24 Hour) Method

This method of fasting is incredibly similar to the crescendo method. The only discernable difference is that there's no anticipation of increasing into a more intense fasting pattern with time. For the eat-stop-eat method, you decide which days you want to take off from eating, and then you run with it until you've lost that weight and then you keep running with the lifestyle for good because you won't be able to imagine life without it.

The eat-stop-eat method involves one to two days a week being

100% oriented towards fasting, with the other five to six days concerning "business as normal." The one or two days spent fasting are then full 24-hour days spent without eating anything at all. During these days, of course, water and coffee are still fine to drink, but no food items can be consumed whatsoever. Exercise is also frowned upon on those fasting days but see what your body can handle before you decide how that should all work out.

Some people might start thinking they're using the crescendo method but end up sticking with eat-stop-eat.

## Alternate-Day Method

The alternate-day method is admittedly a little confusing, but the reason it could be so confusing could come, in part, from how much wiggle room it provides for the practitioner. This method is great for people who don't have a consistent schedule or any sense of one, and it is therefore incredibly forgiving for those who don't quite have everything together for themselves yet.

When it comes down to it, alternate-day intermittent fasting is really up to you. You should try to fast every other day, but it doesn't have to be that precise. Similarly, with crescendo method, as long as you fast two to three days a week, with a break day or two in between each fasting day, you're set! Basically then, you'll want to eat normally for three or four days out of each week, and when you encounter a fasting day, you don't even need to completely fast!

Alternate-day fasting is a solid place to start from, especially if you work a varying schedule or still have yet to get used to a consistent one. If you want to make things more intense from this starting point, the alternate-day method can easily become the eat-stop-eat method, the crescendo method, or the 5:2 method. Essentially, this method is a great place to begin

## 12:12 Method

As another of the more natural ways of intermittent fasting, 12:12 approach is well-suited to beginning practitioners. Many people live out 12:12 method without any forethought simply because of their sleeping and eating schedule but turning 12:12 into a conscious practice can have just as many positive effects on your life as the more drastic 20:4 method claims.

According to a study conducted in the University of Alabama For this method, in particular, you fast for 12 hours and then enter a 12-hour eating window. It's not difficult whatsoever to get three small meals and several snacks, or two big meals and a snack into your day with this method. With 12:12, the standard meal timing works just fine.

Ultimately, this method is a great one to start from, for a lot of variation can be built into this scheduling when you're ready to make things more interesting. Effortlessly and without much effort, 12:12 can become 14:10 or even 16:8, and in seemingly no time, you can find yourself trying alternate-day or crescendo methods, too. Start with what's normal for you, and this method might be exactly that!

## 5:2 Method

This is another popular way to fast, because there is no true fasting involved, but instead a strict and drastic reduction of calories for two days each week. So, for five days a week, you are going to eat your normal 1.600 to 2,000 calories and exercising like normal. The on two nonconsecutive days a week you are going to restrict your caloric intake to between 500 and 600 calories. When doing this pay close attention the number of calories in beverages as well, many people make the mistake of only counting calories in what they eat. Remember, that beverages contain calories too, especially if you are drinking things from coffee shops, as these have a tendency to have high amounts of sugar.

## Crescendo Method

This is usually an introduction to fasting, it is how many people begin their fasting journey. This is a less intense form of intermittent fasting and is a great way for you to see how it works to ease your fears and become familiarized with a fasting schedule. This method involves normally for 4 or 5 days a week and then restricting your eating period to between 8 or 10 hours for two or three nonconsecutive days. Very similar to the 16/8 method, but instead of doing every day, you only do it a couple days each week. These are the safest ways for women to fast because they do not upset the hormonal balance of the body.

Intermittent fasting not done properly can trick the body into going into what is known as starvation mode. This happens when the body thinks it needs to hold onto fat longer because it doesn't know when it will have a chance to consume food for fuel again. This can lead to burning muscle for fuel as well as upsetting the hormonal balance, leading to even more issues. However, intermittent fasting done properly can be safe and incredibly beneficial.

Not only does intermittent fasting help you lose weight, but it also improves mental clarity and allows you to simplify your life in a way that diets do not. Think about how much time you spend worrying about or eating food, and then imagine what other things you could be doing if this were not the case. This is one the major benefits of intermittent fasting, there are no surprises and you are able to take complete control of when you eat.

# Chapter 3: The Need of Intermittent fasting for Woman

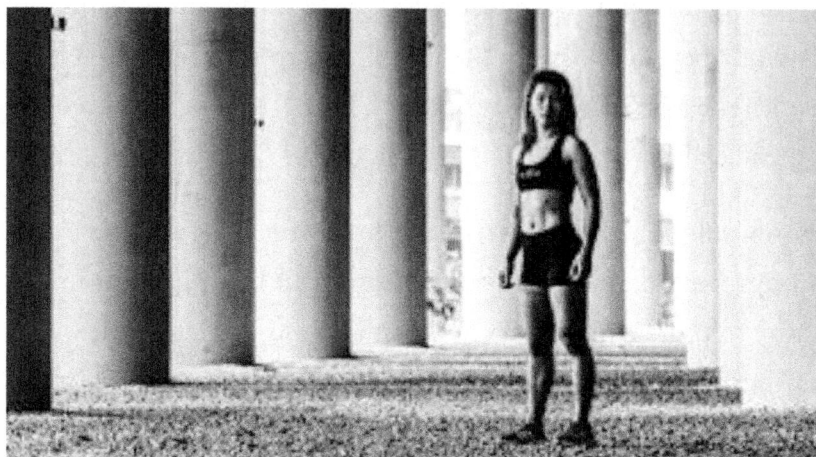

For those interested in losing weight, intermittent fasting may seem like an excellent option. However, many people would like to know if women should fast. Is intermittent fasting reliable for women? There have been a couple of studies of study essential for the intermittent fasting can help you lose weight in this fascinating new food trend. Intermittent fasting is also called alternative daily fasting, although there are some variations in this diet plan. The American Journal of Clinical Nutrition recently conducted a research study that included 16 overweight men and women in a 10-week program. On fasting days, people absorbed food up to 25% of their approximate energy needs. The rest of the time, they received dietary training; however, they were not given a particular criterion to meet during this period. What made this exploration fascinating is that many people need to lose even more weight than those who study the research before seeing the same settings. It was a fantastic discovery that encouraged a large number of people to try fasting. Intermittent fasting for women has some positive results. Women with a healthy diet and training strategy may have problems with persistent fat; However, fasting is a reasonable solution for this.

## Intermittent fasting for women over 50 years.

Without a doubt, our bodies and our metabolic rate change when we reach menopause. One of the most important changes experienced by women over 50 is that they have a slower metabolic process and begin to gain weight. Fasting can be an unusual way to avoid this weight and also change the gain. study

The studies try to show that this model fasting helps control hunger, and people who do not regularly even experience the same aspirations of others. If you are over 50 years old and also try to slow down the metabolic process, recurring fasting can help you stop consuming too much daily. Your body also begins to establish some chronic conditions such as high cholesterol and hypertension when it reaches 50 years. Intermittent fasting has been exposed to reduce cholesterol and blood stress, even without a fantastic offer of weight reduction. If you began to see your numbers improve every year in the doctor's work environment, you might have the opportunity to reduce them on an empty stomach, even without losing much weight. Recurring fasting may not be an exceptional idea for all single women. Anyone with a specific health condition or who often tends to be hypoglycemic should talk to a doctor. This new dietary pattern has special benefits for women who naturally store more fat in their bodies and may also have difficulty getting rid of these fat deposits.

# Chapter 4: What's the Best over 50

We will help you understand how to pick out the right plan when it comes to intermittent fasting protocol. One thing to realize would be that intimate fasting can be customized based on your needs. If you are someone looking to have eating schedules based on your lifestyle, then chances are intermittent fasting is the answer for you. As you know, by now, there are tons of ways for you to follow intermittent fasting. We talked about the different intermittent fasting protocols, and which one will benefit you in what way. One thing to remember is that you will still see many of the benefits we . regardless of the plan you follow. This means that following intermittent fasting or certain protocol should not demotivate you when it comes to following a certain plan.

Now, you have to remember that we can only go through certain lifestyles and scenarios. Don't expect us to have a perfect scenario for you. However, all the scenarios should be close to the scenario you are living in. also, if we suggest a certain intermittent fasting protocol based on the scenarios, make sure that you still try on all the intermittent fasting protocols and realize which one works for you. The truth is, the best personal trainer is the best nutritionist you're going to have you. Once you start understanding your body, then you will be in a much better position of not only utilizing intermittent fasting at its full potential, but you also have a great idea off went to stop and when you should begin.

If that makes sense, then you should be steps ahead of your trainers and nutritionists, which you might hire. We are not saying that you should not have a personal trainer or nutritionist, what we are saying is that you will be in a much better position if you can understand how your body functions to create a customized plan for you. Now the first scenario we are going to be using would be very similar to someone who works in a nine-to-five job. If you're someone who works from 9 to 5 and only gets one lunch break during the day and chances are 16/ 8, intermittent fasting would be ideal for you. To clarify, you can always start with a 12/12 intermittent fasting protocol, in the beginning, to get ready. However, once you get your feet wet with intermittent fasting, then you should go with the 16/8 method.

The reason why the 16/8 method works so well for people who work a 9to five job it is because it is straightforward to manage. The beauty of the 16/8 method when it comes to intermittent fasting is that you can set the hours to whatever time you want to eat, and you don't want to eat. For example, many people notice better brain functioning when they are not eating any food. This means you can skip breakfast and not eat throughout the whole workday allowing you to focus on the task at hand. Then once you're done working, you can have yourself a nice big breakfast. We know numerous amounts of people doing this, and not only did the notice they lost a lot of weight, but they also got a lot better at the work which they are performing. The beauty of intermittent fasting would be that it allows you to not only lose body fat but give you the mental clarity that you're looking for.

The reason why you get mental Clarity is that you will not be spiking up your insulin throughout the day. When you spike up your insulin, you will notice things such as lethargy and overall laziness. This is why the 16/8 method works so great when it comes to recovering any issues which you might be facing when it comes to mental fog or mental fatigue. That being said, start with the 12/12 method and slowly build-up to the 16/8 method to see better results. In this scenario, not only will your work performance go up, but you also lose a lot of weight and get the overall health benefits that you're looking for when it comes to intermittent fasting. This will work especially well for people who are above the age of 50.

The reason why it will work a lot better for people who are above the age of 50 is simply that they will go through a phase known as autophagy. As you know, autophagy has been shown to reduce many health complications, including the slowing down of aging. This makes it ideal for people looking to slow down aging. So if you work a nine-to-five job and you're looking to lose body fat while slowing down aging, then we highly recommend that you follow the 16/8 method throughout the workday. Meaning fastest route to the workday, and have yourself a nice breakfast after you're done working. I want you to perform a lot better at your workplace, and to see better results overall when it comes to intermittent fasting and losing body fat. Keep in mind, the scenario we just talked about is the first scenario that most people will be going through.

However, we have a ton of scenarios to talk about. Now chances are there will be a lot of people who work in labor, looking to reap the benefits of intermittent fasting. Now, if you are working labor, chances are it will be a little bit more difficult for you to continue with intermittent passing. However, with the right scheduling in the right planning, you should have no problem concerning intermittent fasting. Now let's say you work the labor 8 hours a day. What we would recommend is trying to have most of your calories throughout the 8-hour window. Once you are done with your work, make sure that you start your fast right away.

Now there are a lot of ways for you to get your calories throughout your eating window while you are working. You can have things such as protein shake, and You are quickly you going to have a pre-prepared meal, which will help you to consume all the calories you need throughout the whole day. The reason why we recommend you eat throughout the day while you're working is that a labor job could be tedious. We want to make sure that you don't paint or affect your work in any way possible. This is why we recommend you follow the 16 by eight method and include your eating window while you are working. Many people who work in labor tend to follow this protocol, the reason why it works so well. That's because they won't get all the calories they need when they need it. You need to have a good steady flow of food intake while you are physically working.

Your body can only break down fat so quickly, which is why a good amount of carbohydrates and nutrients is important when you're performing anything physical. That being said, you can always resort to the 5/2 method when you are intermittent fasting. If you don't like the 16/8 method, then you can always follow the 5/2 method. This method works great as you only have to "fast" for two days out of the week, meaning you can normally eat when you are working. As you get older, especially in the labor workforce, you will be required to be well-fed when you're working. The last thing we want is for you to have injuries at your workplace. That being said, you can either follow the 16/8 method, or you can go right ahead and follow the 5/2 method fasting on your non-working days.

This will allow you to see the results that you're looking for when it comes to anti-aging, regardless of the fasting protocol you follow. However, if we're honest, the 16/8 method works a lot better when it comes to seeing results in regards to intermittent fasting and anti-aging. Now let's pick out another scenario, what's talked about someone who works the night shift. If you're someone who works the night shift, the chances are that you will be in a much better scenario than a lot of people. The reason why you will be in a much better position than a lot of people are that nightshift tends to be slow for most cases. Now, if you're a nurse, then chances are you will have no time to eat any food.

So the best thing for you to do would be not to have any food during your shift, and once you're done your shift, you can have more food allowing you to be a lot better at fasting. The great thing about being a nurse or working a night shift would be that you will have a much better position of not only continued with intermittent fasting but the desire to not eat. Numerous times we have heard nurses talk about not having the time to eat, or simply not in the mood for eating anything. Having this mentality will help you tremendously to continue with intermittent fasting, which is why it is so important to understand which intermittent fasting protocol works for your needs. Batting said if your nurse is working night shifts, the best-case scenario for you would be too fast brought your whole shift and have your eating window once you're done your work. For instance, let's say you work 10 hours a day, then fast for 10 hours a day and eat for the remainder of the time. This gets a little bit tricky for a nurse, as the hours can be scattered or sometimes not be ideal case scenario for you too fast. However, the best way to go about fasting if your nurse who is who works a shift at a very demanding job, we recommend you fast during the time you are working. This will allow you to be in a perfect position when it comes to fasting and to see the best results overall with intermittent fasting. In essence, you will be trying out all the types of intermittent fasting when you are working the night shift or working as a nurse, for example. Depending on your shift, you will be fasting either 10 hours or even up to 24 hours, depending on how you feel. That being said, this will give you the best possible scenario for you to continue with intermittent fasting and to make it a habit. Many people don't realize it, but making intermittent fasting a part of your life is much more important than someone looking to follow a specific plan. Now we have given you enough scenarios to figure out which plan would work best for you based on your lifestyle. Now we will move on and talk about all the methods and which deliver the specific goal that you're looking for. Keep in mind that all these plans will work tremendously well if you're looking to slow down aging and to lose body fat overall feeling better about yourself. However, we will break down all the plans so that you have a better idea of which one to pick and finalize.

16/8: As you know, the 16/8 method is one of the most popular ways when it comes to intermittent fasting. The 16/8 way will not only help you to lose body fat, but it will also help you with the anti-aging process and to better your overall function. Many people follow the 16/8 method as it is the most convenient method to follow and comfortably flexible. Depending on your lifestyle, this method could work very well when it comes to giving you the results that you're looking for. The beauty of this method is that you can build muscle, lose fat, and do anything you want while making this a life choice. When I say a life choice, it means that you can follow this plan for the rest of your life and not feel taxed out. If it is feasible for you, then we highly recommend that you follow the 16/8 method, one of the most studied ways of intermittent fasting.

12/12: Now, this method is for someone who's looking to set up intermittent fasting without going too hard if you don't know how intermittent fasting works or you don't know if it is going to be the right path for you then you should start with the 12/12 method. This method will allow you to get your feet wet when it comes to intermittent fasting so that you can continue with intermittent fasting if you enjoy it or make it a little bit more challenging by upping the fasting times. That being said, but

12/12 method is merely something to get your feet wet with and not something you should do for the rest of your life. The secure trolls method is a great plan to start. However, you will not see the anti-aging effects or the weight loss effects that you're looking for following this method. In the beginning, you will, however, as you go along, you will not see the results that you are looking for when it comes to losing body fat are slowing down the aging process. This is where the 16/8 method will shine, as it will give you sufficient time to fast while seeing the benefits that you are hoping to get out of intermittent fasting.

The water fast: Now the water fast is for someone who is looking to not only detoxify their body, but they're changing the way their body functions. This plan is only to be followed a handful of times to detoxify their gut, so they digest a lot better. If you might know, the stomach is known as the second brain. The reason why it is known as a second brain is that your body heavily depends on your gut and how it digests, as you know, eating food as necessary for a livelihood, which is why we must take care of the organs, especially our gut. Make sure you use this method to clean out your organs and to see better results from it. This will allow you to be in a better position when it comes to digesting food and keeping your organs beautiful and safe.

5:2 Diet: This fasting protocol is ideal for people who are looking to lose weight quickly, now if you're someone who wants to lose weight rapidly and has a motivation and willpower to get it done then the 5/2 works the best. A disciple makes you lose a lot of body fat and a short period, allowing you to live a lot better life overall. Now keep in mind that following the 5/2 diet will not help you with any anti-aging process in the long-term. But I will help you detoxify your body and to make you lose a ton of weight, especially in the beginning. Don't follow this protocol for the rest of your life as it is not sustainable. However, once you get the hang of this plan, you will be in a much better position to lose fat and to get your goal weight a lot quicker than you would. Once you've lost a way to find the 5/2 diet, we recommend that you started following the 16/8 diet quickly. The 16/8 diet is where you want to be when it comes to seeing long-lasting results. Regardless of the 5/2 diet will work for you if you do a labor job, because of the structure.

Keep in mind that we want you to use your brain when it comes to picking out the right plan. As always, make sure that you know your body before you start following any of these plans. We recommend a start off with a 12/12 method as you will see significant benefits from it in the beginning. However, once you get your feet wet with intermittent fasting, then we recommend that you start following other plans that will help you achieve that goal as well.

# Chapter 5: The Benefits of Intermittent Fasting

## Weight loss

Intermittent Fasting switches from periods of eating and to periods of fasting. If you fast, naturally, your calorie intake will reduce, and it also helps you maintain your weight loss. It also prevents you from indulging in mindless eating. Whenever you eat something, your body converts the food into glucose and fat. It uses this glucose immediately and stores the fat for later use. When you skip a few meals, your body starts to reach into its internal stores of fat to provide energy. As soon as the body begins burning fats due to the shortage of glucose, you will start to lose weight. Also, most of the fat that you lose is from the abdominal region. If you want a flat tummy, then this is the perfect diet for you.

## Tackles diabetes

Diabetes is a significant threat on its own. It is also a primary indicator of the increase in risk factors of various cardiovascular diseases like heart attacks and strokes. When the glucose level increases alarmingly in the bloodstream, and there isn't enough insulin to process this glucose, it causes diabetes. When your body resists insulin, it becomes difficult to regulate insulin levels in the body. Intermittent Fasting reduces insulin sensitivity and helps tackle diabetes.

## Sleep

Lack of sleep is one of the main causes of obesity. When your body doesn't get enough sleep, the internal mechanism of burning fat suffers. Intermittent Fasting regulates your sleep cycle and, in turn, makes your body effectively burn fats. A good sleep cycle has different physiological benefits - it makes you feel energetic and elevates your overall mood.

### Resistance to illnesses

Intermittent Fasting helps in the growth and regeneration of cells. Did you know that the human body has an internal mechanism that helps repair damaged cells? Intermittent Fasting helps kickstart this mechanism. It improves the overall functioning of all the cells in the body. So, it is directly responsible for improving your body's natural defense mechanism by increasing its resistance to diseases and illnesses.

### A healthy heart

Intermittent Fasting assists in weight loss, and weight loss improves your cardiovascular health. A buildup of plaque in blood vessels is known as atherosclerosis. This is the primary cause of various cardiovascular diseases. The endothelium is the thin lining of blood vessels, and any dysfunction in it results in atherosclerosis. Obesity is the primary problem that plagues humanity and is also the main reason for the increase of plaque deposits in the blood vessels. Stress and inflammation also increase the severity of this problem. Intermittent Fasting tackles the buildup of fat and helps tackle obesity. So, all you need to do is follow the simple protocols of Intermittent Fasting to improve your overall health.

### A healthy gut

There are several millions of microorganisms present in your digestive system. These microorganisms help improve the overall functioning of your digestive system and are known as the gut microbiome. Intermittent Fasting enhances the health of these microbiomes and improves your digestive health. A healthy digestive system helps in better absorption of food and improves the functioning of your stomach.

### Reduces inflammation

Whenever your body feels there is an internal problem, its natural defense is inflammation. It doesn't mean that all forms of inflammation are desirable. Inflammation can cause several serious health conditions like arthritis, atherosclerosis, and other neurodegenerative disorders.

Any inflammation of this nature is known as chronic inflammation and is quite painful. Chronic inflammation can restrict your body's movements too. If you want to keep inflammation in check, then Intermittent Fasting will certainly come in handy.

### Promotes cell repair

When you fast, the cells in your body start the process of waste removal. Waste removal means the breaking down of all dysfunctional cells and proteins and is known as autophagy. Autophagy offers protection against several degenerative diseases like Alzheimer's and cancer. You don't like accumulating garbage in your home, do you? Similarly, your body must not hold onto any unnecessary toxins. Autophagy is the body's way of getting rid of all things useless.

When subjected to food scarcity for a long time, mammals, including humans, will start to experience a decrease in their organ size. One of these organs is the brain. While some organs return to their original size over time, others may be impacted over the long term.

The brain handles the basic cognitive function of the body. In order to function properly and get the needed nutrients, it needs to return to its original size. However, if the brain becomes too foggy, getting the needed food nutrients will be pretty difficult, which might lead to malnutrition and even be fatal. However, during a shorter period of food scarcity, the brain becomes hyperactive in its search for food as a mechanism for survival.

Excessive availability of food and eating altogether makes us mentally dull. Reflect on a time when you were completely satisfied after a big meal. After eating a massive plate of food, you will likely go into a "food coma" and curl up and sleep, or maybe just watch your favorite TV show on Netflix rather than get the motivation to go achieve your goals. Without a doubt, satisfaction from food makes man naturally lose the drive to pursue his goals, which ultimately leads to dulling the brain. With this in mind, know that when you fast, your cognitive abilities are quickened. This improves your mental keenness, allowing you to achieve your health-related goals as opposed to excessively feeding.

It should be established here that there is no scientific research to support the notion that intermittent fasting alters mental alertness negatively. Fasting will not affect your cognitive function, such as moods, mental alertness, reaction time, intention, and sleep in any bad way. On the contrary, these things get boosted during fasting.

This is one of the many wondrous benefits of intermittent fasting, which many people should look forward to. Fasting is amazing in that it keeps the brains cell from degeneration. This is because fasting prevents neural death.

Besides, fasting also triggers the process of autophagy in the brain – autophagy is the process in which the body gets rid of damaged body cells and brings out new ones. When the body is full of healthy, active, and improved cells, it is strong and well-equipped to combat any diseases that might want to attack.

With autophagy, the risk of viral infection, as well as duplication of intracellular parasites, reduces drastically. This dramatically reduces intracellular pathogens, such as cancer cells. Besides, the brain and other body tissue cells are protected from abnormal growth, inflammation, and toxicity.

## Reduced Risk of Depression

With intermittent fasting, there is an increase in the levels of a neurotransmitter called a neurotrophic factor. When the body is deficient in this brain-derived factor, it contributes to significant issues such as depression and other mood disorders. Hence, intermittent fasting is really helpful in improving mental alertness and enhancing mood, which ultimately leads to a reduced tendency to develop these conditions.

There are a couple of metabolic features that get triggered when we fast that improve brain health. This explains why people who practice intermittent fasting do have lower levels of inflammation, low blood sugar levels, and reduced oxidative stress.

There are also indications that intermittent fasting can keep the brain protected against the risk of stroke.

### Intermittent Fasting Fosters Immune Regulation

When you fast, part of the primary aim of the body is to keep the immune system healthy. This is why we encourage drinking a large quantity of water during the period of the intermittent fast, and afterward as well. Water can be spiced up with other detox agents that remove toxins from the digestive system and reduces the number of unhealthy gut microbes. Have in mind that the number of gut microbes present in the gastrointestinal tract is directly related to the immune system's function.

Intermittent fasting determines the number of inflammatory cytokines that the body has. Hence, it helps regulate the body's overall immune system. In the body, we have two significant cytokines that cause inflammation in the body: Interleukin-6 and Tumor Necrosis Factor Alpha. Fasting suppresses the release of these inflammatory pro-inflammatory cytokines.

### Intermittent Fasting Reduces the Risk of Chronic Disease

People living with chronic autoimmune diseases like Crohn's disease, colitis, rheumatoid arthritis, and systemic lupus will definitely see remarkable improvement with intermittent fasting. The idea is simple. Fasting reduces the rate of an extreme inflammatory process in the bodies of these persons. With this, they have an ideal immune function.

For instance, cancer cells have between ten and seventy extra insulin receptors in contrast to healthy body cells. This happens as a result of the breakdown of sugar for fuel. With intermittent fasting, cancer cells are starved of sugar intake. This conditions the cells for damage through free radicals.

The tendency of the body to live longer increases when it does not get enough food. This is because, with intermittent fasting, there is repair and regeneration of cells that come about via a repair mechanism in the body. This is understandable, as the energy required for cell repair is lesser when compared to what is necessary for cell creation or division.

Hence, during the period of intermittent fasting, cell division, and creation in the body becomes reduced. This is a necessary process, vital especially for the healing of malignant cells, which thrive as a result of abnormal cell division.

In the body, the human growth hormone (HGH) takes care of the process of cell repair. It is a human growth hormone that brings about changes in metabolism that cause tissue repair and fat burning. Thus, when we fast, the body can concentrate more on repairing body tissues with amino acids and enzymes. This restores tissue collagen and also triggers an improvement in bones, ligaments, tendons, and the general muscle function in the body.

# Cancer

Lastly, studies have found that intermittent can reduce your likelihood of developing cancer and help make treatment more successful. As you are aware, intermittent fasting can help treat oxidative stress and cellular damage, both of which cause cancer. By reducing this damage, you can thereby reduce your risk of developing cancer in the future.

But that is not all. While human studies still need to be conducted, a study on mice found that when practicing short-term fasting chemotherapy treatment becomes more successful in targeting and treating both breast cancer and skin cancer. Not only did the chemotherapy itself become more effective, but the mice' immune systems also were better able to fight off the cancerous cells and growths, which is essential as chemotherapy is well-known for reducing a person's immune system drastically.

# Chapter 6: Intermittent Fasting Potential Downsides

## Anxiety Attacks

Another potential side effect of detoxing through intermittent fasting is the potential for an anxiety attack. This can happen when you are withholding food for an extended period of time especially if you are new to intermittent fasting.

An anxiety attack may come upon because you feel that you are not getting enough nutrition, or you are missing your usual feeding times.

## Digestive Distress

Since intermittent fasting has a detoxing component to it, you may experience digestive distress during your first few experiences. This is due to your body flushing out much of the residual matter in your body in addition to simply excreting whatever is still left over in the digestive tract.

While this is normal to a certain extent, care should be taken if you happen to experience severe diarrhea. This may be especially true if you jump into a fasting period after overeating the previous day. As long as it isn't anything that you feel to be abnormal, then you can attribute it to the detoxing process. However, if symptoms do not subside then you may need to seek medical attention at once.

# You Might Struggle to Maintain Blood Sugar Levels

Although the intermittent fasting diet tends to improve blood sugar levels in most people, this is not always true for everyone. Some people who are eating following the intermittent fasting diet may find that their ability to maintain a healthy blood sugar level is compromised.

The reason for why this happens varies. For some people, not eating frequently enough may encourage this to happen. For others, transitioning too quickly or taking on too intense of a fasting cycle too soon can result in a shock to the body that causes a strange fluctuation in blood sugar levels.

# You Might Experience Hormonal Imbalances

A certain degree of fasting, especially when you build up to it, can support you in having healthier hormone levels. However, for some people, intermittent fasting may lead to an unhealthy imbalance of hormones. This can result in a whole slew of different hormone-based symptoms, such as headaches, fatigue, and even menstrual problems in women.

Again, the reason for the hormonal imbalance varies. For some people, particularly those who are already at risk of experiencing hormonal imbalances, intermittent fasting can trigger these imbalances to take place. For others, it could go back to what they are consuming during the eating windows. Eating meals that are not rich in nutrients and vitamins can result in you not having enough nutrition to support your hormonal levels.

If you begin experiencing hormonal imbalances when you eat the intermittent fasting diet, it is essential that you stop and consult your doctor right away. Discovering where the shortcomings are and how you can correct them is vital. Having imbalanced hormones for too long can lead to diseases and illnesses that require constant life-long attention.

## Headaches

A decrease in your blood sugar level and the release of stress hormones by your brain as a result of going without food are possible causes of headaches during the fasting window. Problems may also be a clear message from your body telling you that you are very low on water and getting dehydrated. This may happen if you are completely engrossed in your daily activities, and you forget to drink the required amount of water your body needs during fasting.

To handle headaches, ensure you stay well hydrated throughout your fasting window. Keep in mind that exceeding the required amount of water per day may also result in adverse effects. Reducing your stress level can also keep headaches away.

## Cravings

During your fasting periods, you might find that you have higher levels of desires than usual. This often happens because you are telling yourself that you cannot have any food, so suddenly you start craving many different foods. This is because all you are thinking about is food. As you think about food, you will begin to think about the different types of food that you like and that you want. Then, the cravings start.

Early on, you may also find yourself craving more sweets or carbs because your body is searching for an energy hit through glucose. While you do not want to have excessive levels of sugar during your eating window, as this is bad for blood sugar, you can always have some. The ability to satisfy your cravings is one of the benefits of eating a diet that is not as restrictive as some other foods are.

## Low Energy

A feeling of lethargy is not uncommon during fasting, especially at the start. This is your body's natural reaction to switching its source of energy from glucose in your meals to fat stored in your body. So, expect to feel a little less energized in your first few weeks of starting with intermittent fasting. To troubleshoot the feeling of lethargy, try as much as possible to stay away from overly strenuous activities. Keep things low key. Spending more time sleeping or just relaxing is another right way to ensure that your energy reserves are not depleted too quickly. The first few weeks are not the time to test your limits or push yourself.

## Foul Mood

You may find yourself being on edge during fasting, even if you are someone who is naturally predisposed to being good-natured. The reason for the feeling of edginess is straightforward. You are hungry, yet you won't eat, and you are struggling to keep your cravings in check, plus, you may already be feeling tired and sluggish. Add all of these to the internal hormone changes due to the sharp decline in your blood sugar levels, and it's no wonder why you may be in such a foul mood. Tempers can easily flare up, and you may be quick to become irritated. This is normal when beginning a fasting lifestyle.

## Excess Urination

Fasting tends to make you visit the bathroom more frequently than usual. This is an expected side effect since you are drinking more water and other liquids than before. Avoiding water to reduce the number of times you use the bathroom is not a good idea at all, no matter how you look at it. Cutting down water intake while you are fasting will make your body become dehydrated very quickly. If that happens, losing weight will be the least of your problems. Whatever you do, do not avoid drinking water when you are fasting. Doing that is paving the way for a humongous health disaster waiting to happen. You don't want to do that.

## Heartburn, Bloating, and Constipation

Your stomach is responsible for producing stomach acid, which is used to break down food and trigger the digestion process. When you eat frequent meals, unusually large meals, regularly, your body is used to producing high amounts of stomach acid to break down your food. As you transition to a fasting diet, your stomach has to get used to not producing as much stomach acid.

You might also notice an increase in constipation and bloating. People who eat regularly consume high amounts of fiber and proteins that support a healthy digestion process. When you switch to the intermittent fasting cycle, you can still eat a high volume of fiber and protein. However, early on, you might find that you forget to. As you discover the right eating habits that work for you, it may take some time for you to get used to finding ways to work in enough fiber and protein to keep your digestion flowing.

Heartburn may not be a widespread adverse effect, but it does sometimes occur in some individuals. Your stomach produces highly concentrated acids to help break down the foods you consume. But when you are fasting, there is no food in your stomach to be broken down, even though acids have already been produced for that purpose. This may lead to heartburn.

Bloating and constipation usually go hand in hand and can be very discomforting to individuals who suffer from it due to fasting.

Heeding the advice to drink adequate amounts of water usually keeps bloating and constipation in check. Heartburn typically resolves itself quickly, but you can take an antacid tablet or two if it persists. You may also consider eating fewer spicy foods when you break your fast.

# You Might Experience Low Energy and Irritability

Until now, your body has been used to having a constant stream of energy pouring in all day long. From the time you wake up until the time you go to bed, it has been receiving some form of power from the foods that you eat. So, when you stop eating regularly, your body grows confused. It has to learn to create its energy rather than rely on the heat being offered to it by the food that you are eating.

Depending on how you are eating, your body may also be growing used to consuming fat as a fuel source rather than carbohydrates. This means that, in addition to losing its primary energy source, it also has to switch how it consumes energy and where it comes from. This can lead to lowered energy for a while. Do things that exert the least amount of energy. If you are someone who regularly exercises and works out, reducing the amount that you work out or switching to a more relaxed workout like yoga can help you during the transition period.

## You Might Start Feeling Cold

As you begin to adjust to your intermittent fasting diet, you might find that your fingers and toes get quite cold. This happens because blood flow towards your fat stores is increasing, so blood flow to your extremities reduces slightly. This supports your body in moving fat to your muscles so that it can be burned as a fuel to keep your energy levels up.

## You Might Find Yourself Overeating

The chances for overeating during the break of the fast are high, especially for beginners. Understandably, you will feel starving after going without food for longer than you are used to. It is this hunger that causes some people to eat hurriedly and surpass their standard meal size and average caloric intake. For others, overeating may be as a result of uncontrollable appetite. Hunger may push some people to prepare too much food for breaking their fast, and if they don't have a grip on their desire, they will continue to eat even when they are satiated. Overeating or binging when you break your fast will make it difficult to reach your goal of optimal health and fitness.

## Hunger Pangs

People who start intermittent fasting may initially feel quite hungry. This is especially common if you are the type of person who tends to eat regular meals daily.

If you start feeling hungry, you can choose to wait it out if you have an eating window right around the corner. However, if there is a more extended waiting period or you are feeling excessively hungry, you should eat. Feeling hungry to the point that it becomes uncomfortable or distracting is not helpful and will not support you in successfully taking on the intermittent fasting diet. This is a pronounced side effect of going without food for longer than you are accustomed to.

## Headaches

One other symptom that may affect you during fasting is a headache. This is a natural reaction by the brain to the sudden change in chemical composition as a result of the detoxing process. You may find that you get a slight headache which will go away on its own.

However, a strong headache and persistent headache may be a side effect of the detoxing process or just a lack of food. Since you have an empty stomach, taking headache medication would be ill-advised as it may trigger digestive distress. If your headache is unbearable, then you may need to have food with the medication.

# Chapter 7: Is The Intermittent Fasting For Everyone?

There are excellent bargains of various diet plans that you can pick from. Some help you limit your carb intake and focus on the great fats and healthy proteins. Some will restrict your fat consumption and also concentrate on healthy and balanced and superb carbs.

With all the alternatives in the industry, and with at least a few of them being reputable selections for lowering weight, you might ask yourself why you must choose Intermittent fasting. This phase will have a look at the various benefits of periodic fasting and also how it will make a distinction in your health.

**Change the feature of cells, hormones, and genetics**

Numerous things take place to your body when you do not consume for some time. Your body will start initiating procedures for cell repair work as well as alteration some of your hormonal agent degrees, which makes maintained body fat much easier to obtain accessibility to.

Other adjustments that can occur in the body contain: Insulin degrees: Your insulin degrees will come by a reasonable bit, which makes it easier for the body to melt fat

Human development hormone agent: The blood levels of the development hormonal agent can significantly raise. Greater levels of this hormonal representative can assist construct muscular tissue as well as burn fat.

Mobile repair work: The body will certainly begin important

mobile repair procedures, such as getting rid of all the waste from cells.

Gene expression: Some helpful modifications happen in countless genetics that will assist you to live longer and also secure against disease.

## Drop weight and body fat.

Lots of people go on an Intermittent quick to go down weight. Essentially, Intermittent fasting will naturally help you in consuming fewer meals. You will certainly wind up absorbing fewer calories, which will result in weight reduction.

Fasting improves the hormone feature to assist with weight-loss. Greater development hormone levels, as well as reduced insulin, assist your body to break down fat as well as utilize it for energy. This is why short-term fasting can boost your metabolic process by a minimum of 3 percent.

On one hand, it enhances your metabolic rate to make certain that you burn a lot of extra calories while likewise minimizing just how much you eat. According to a 2014 evaluation of specialist research study on intermittent fasting, people could lose up to 8percent of their body weight in much less than 24 weeks.

Helps with diabetes

Type-2 diabetes is an illness that has ended up being substantial in current decades. Anything that minimizes your insulin resistance needs to help decrease your blood glucose levels and also secure you versus kind 2 diabetes mellitus. Some researches show exactly how

Periodic fasting can have a benefit in insulin resistance and also can help create an amazing reduction in blood glucose levels.

In several research studies on Intermittent fasting, blood glucose was lowered by three to six percent, while insulin level was reduced by twenty to thirty-one percent. One research study on diabetic person rats also revealed that periodic fasting might secure the rat against kidney damages, which is a typical issue with a lot more extreme kinds of diabetes. This reveals that recurring fasting could be an outstanding option for anyone with a higher hazard of establishing type-2 diabetic issues.

There are some differences between the genders. There is one research that disclosed that for females, blood glucose level control might worsen after taking place the periodic fast for a couple of weeks. It's advisable to talk to your doctor before starting any type of diet plan.

## Streamlines life

While this may not be considered a wellness advantage like the others, it is still a crucial one to point out. Great deals of individuals discover that intermittent fasting can make their lives less complex. They figure out that they do not require focusing way too much on the calories they are eating, as long as they remain within the hours that they are allowed to eat. They can go a few days a week without requiring fretting about making a meal. Generally, this diet regimen plan can make your life less complicated.

When you can reduce out a few of the jobs that you require doing throughout the day and emphasize another thing, you can end up with less stress and anxiety in your life. All of us understand just how extreme stress can have a negative impact on our wellness and life. When you can reduce stress, it is a lot simpler to be the healthiest variation of yourself.

Can aid with cancer

Several individuals have cancer cells yearly. The unchecked advancement of cells defines this horrible condition. Fasting has been disclosed to have some outstanding benefits when it pertains to your metabolic process, which may cause a lowered threat of cancer cells.

Some human research study studies disclose that cancer cells customers who fasted could lessen a few of the side results that include chemotherapy.

## Useful for the mind

What is thought of fantastic for the body advantages the mind likewise? Intermittent fasting can help improve metabolic functions that are comprehended for aiding the mind to stay healthy. This could include assisting with insulin resistance, blood sugar level decrease, lowered inflammation, and oxidative tension.

There have actually been some research study studies done on rats that demonstrate just how intermittent fasting can aid boost the development of brand-new afferent nerve cells, which improves the mind's function. Not eating can likewise assist in boosting the degrees of the brain-derived neurotrophic aspect. When the brain is lacking in this, it can activate depression together with a few other mind worries.

## Assists with cellular fixing

The cells in the body can start a waste removal when we go on a quick process that is recognized as autophagy which involves the cells breaking down and metabolizing any kind of healthy proteins that can not be made use of any kind of longer. With an increased amount of autophagy, it might help guard the body versus diseases such as Alzheimer's and also cancer cells.

## May prevent Alzheimer

Alzheimer is amongst the most common neurodegenerative illness. There is no cure for Alzheimer's, so the best step is to prevent it from happening as much as possible. One study that was carried out on rats showed that Intermittent fasting could be able to delay the start of Alzheimer illness or minimize the intensity of it.

Some reports have really shown that a way of life modification that included some daily, or a minimum of regular, temporary fasts aided to improve the signs of Alzheimer's in 9 out of 10 clients. Pet research study studies additionally expose that this kind of fasting may aid in safeguarding against various other neurodegenerative diseases, such as Huntington's illness and Parkinson's.

Intermittent fasting is a pattern, and research studies on ways it makes your body healthier are sensibly brand-new. It will invest some time to examine all the advantages of recurring fasting.

## Intermittent Fasting can help you in living much longer.

Amongst one of the most interesting attributes of periodic fasting is that it can assist you to live longer. There have actually been several research studies of rats that demonstrated exactly how.

Intermittent fasting may help prolong their life-span - comparable to what takes place when you take place a constant calorie limitation. In some research study studies, the impacts were amazing. In one of them, when the rats did not ate every other day, they end up living 83 percent longer than the rats that didn't go fasting.

It has truly been tough to reveal an increase in life-span due to the fact that periodic fasting has yet to be analyzed on people adequate time to identify this, it is still a prominent concept for those who are trying to stop aging. Offered that there are recognized benefits to metabolic price with this diet regimen, it is not uncommon that individuals think that Intermittent fasting will certainly able to help them live much longer, and likewise much healthier lives.

As you can see, there are big amounts of benefits of choosing the repeating fasting diet regimen. We simply reviewed a few of them, however, there have actually been many research study studies done on the results of this diet plan as well as why it can benefit you. Whether you are attempting to boost brain health, live a lot longer, drop weight, or obtain even more power.

Periodic fasting can boost your life. It does not have any one of these drawbacks.

# Chapter 8: Foods to Enjoy/Avoid

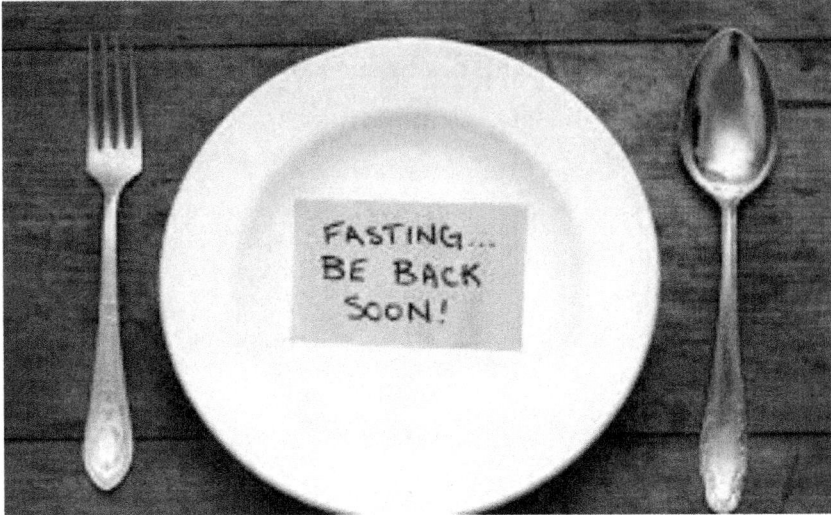

## Foods to Eat

- Eggs - Make sure you eat the yolk because this contains the vitamins Nd protein!

- Leafy greens - We're talking about things like spinach, collards, Kale, and Swiss chards to name a few, and these are packed with fiber and low in calories too

- Oily and fatty fish, such as salmon - Salmon is a fish which will keep you feeling full, but it's also high in omega 3 fatty acids which are ideal for boosting brain health, reducing inflammation, and generally helping with weight loss too. If salmon isn't your bag, try mackerel, trout, herring, and sardines instead

- Cruciferous vegetables - In this case, you need to look toward Brussels sprouts, broccoli, cabbage, and cauliflower. Again, these types of vegetables contain a high fiber amount which helps you feel fuller for longer, but also have cancer-fighting attributes

- Lean meats - Stick to beef and chicken for the best options, but make sure that you go for the leanest cuts possible. You'll get a good protein boost here, but you can also make all manner of delicious dishes with both types of meat!

- Boiled potatoes - You might think that potatoes are bad for you, and in most cases, they are, especially if you fry them, but boiled potatoes are actually a good choice, especially if you lack in potassium. They are also very filling.

- Tuna - This is a different type of fish to the oily fish we mentioned earlier, and it's very low fat, but high in protein. Go for tuna which is canned containing water and not oil for the healthiest option. Pile it onto a jacket potato for a delicious and healthy meal!

- Beans and other types of legumes - These are the staple of any healthy diet and are super filling too. We're talking about things like kidney beans, lentils' Nd black beans here, and they're high in fiber and protein.

- Cottage cheese - If you're a cheese fan, there's no reason to deny yourself, but most cheeses are quite high in fat. In that case, why not opt for cottage cheese instead? This is high in protein and quite filling, but low in calories.

- Avocados - The fad food of the moment is actually very healthy and great for boosting your brain power! Mash it up on some toast for a great breakfast packed with potassium and plenty of fiber.

- Nuts - Instead of snacking on chocolate and crisps, why not snack on nuts? You'll get great amounts of healthy fats, as well as fiber and protein, and they're filling too. Don't eat too many, however, as they can be high in calories if you overindulge.

- Whole grains - Everyone knows that whole grains are packed with fiber and therefore keep you fuller for longer, so this is the ideal choice for anyone who is trying intermittent fasting. Try quinoa, brown rice, and oats to get you started.

- Fruits - Not all fruits are healthy, but they're certainly a better option than chocolate and crisps! You'll also get a plethora of different vitamins and minerals, as well as a boost of antioxidants into your diet - ideal for your immune system.

- Seeds - Again, just like nuts, seeds make a great snack, and they can be sprinkled on many foods, such as yogurt and porridge. Try chia seeds for a high fiber treat, whilst being low calorie at the same time.

- Coconut oil and extra virgin olive oil - You will no doubt have heard of the wonders of coconut oil, and this is a very healthy oil to try cooking with. Coconut oil is made up of something called medium-chain triglycerides, and whilst you might panic at the word triglycerides, these are actually the healthy type! If you want to go for something totally low in calories; however, then you can't beat extra virgin olive oil.

- Yogurt - Perfect for a gut health boost, yogurt is your friend because it will keep you full and it also has probiotic content, provided you go for products which say 'live and active cultures' on the pot. Avoid the overly sugary yogurt treats and anything which says 'low fat' normally isn't as positive as it sounds!

Foods to Avoid

- Sugary foods may curb your appetite, but they won't do anything good for your body in the long run. Steer clear for your future ease.

- Highly GMO foods are also things to avoid when you're working through your fast. They can offset the actual nutrition being provided by other foods in your diet.

Drinks to Take

You are allowed to take drinks while fasting. Go for drinks that are nutritious because they are good for the body. Some of the drinks that you can take are listed below;

Water with fruit or veggie slices will provide nourishment and flavor for those times when you're fasting and need a little extra boost!

Probiotic drinks like kombucha or kefir will work to heal your gut and tide you over till the next eating window.

Black coffee will become your new best friend but be sure not to add cream and sugar! They detract from the good work coffee can do for your body during IF.

Teas of any kind are soothing as well as healing for various elements of the body, mind, and soul. Once again, be sure to omit the cream and sugar!

Chilled or heated broths made from vegetables, bone, or animals can sustain one's energy during times of fast, too.

Apple Cider Vinegar shots are great for the tummy and for healing overall! Hippocrates' remedy for any ailment included this and a healthy regimen of fasting occasionally, so you're sure to succeed with this trick.

Water with salt can provide electrolytes, hydration, and brief sustenance for anyone whose stomachs won't stop grumbling.

Fresh-pressed juices are always great for the body, mind, and soul, and in times of IF, they can sustain one's energy and mood during day-long fast periods, in particular.

Wheatgrass shots are just as healthy as ACV shots, with a

whole other subset of benefits. To awaken your body and give a jolt to your system, try these on for size.

Coconut water is more hydrating than standard water, and it's full of additional nutrients, too! Try this alternative if you need some enhancement to your usual water.

## Monitor & Assess Progress

If you are starting intermittent fasting to not only improve your health, but to also lose weight it is very important to take your initial weight, take measurements, and take pictures before you begin.

Scale Weigh-Ins

The morning of day 1 it is important to get on the scale either nude or in very little clothes. It is important to weigh yourself before eating or drinking anything. Choose a time and weigh yourself, this will be known as your starting weight. It is important that you not only weigh yourself but to also write this number down and/or enter it into your phone or an app that you are using to keep track of your progress. I think it's better for you to write it down in a journal along the way so you can see your progress in real time side by side.

It may also be a good idea to calculate your Body Mass Index (BMI) and your Body Fat Percentage, there are apps to calculate both, or a simple google search can result in free calculators to get this information. To prevent my scale victories from being non-victories, I choose the same day and time to weigh myself, once a week, only once a week. While intermittent fasting, you will lose inches faster than you will lose pounds from the scale, it is very important that you understand that, so that you don't get discouraged and quit. Therefore, I recommend to not only weigh yourself but to also take measurements and pictures to always see what progress you have made.

## Measurement Tracking

The morning of day 1 it is important to take your measurements. You will need to buy a measuring tape to have on hand. I purchased one in my favorite color to make me feel better about myself while taking the measurements. It is important to measure yourself before eating or drinking anything. Choose a time and measure yourself, this will be known as your starting measurements. It is important that you not only measure yourself but to also write these numbers down and/or enter it into your phone or an app that you are using to keep track of your progress. I think it's better for you to write it down in a journal along the way so you can see your progress in real time side by side.

I usually take the following measurements: neck circumference, waist, hips, arms, thigh, bust, belly pouch, and calf. You can measure more or less. I take 3 separate measurements from my waist and stomach area, because feel like its 3 separate body parts. I take measurements at the same time each day and week that I weigh myself.

Before & After

The morning of day 1 it is important to take before pictures, so you have proof of how you looked on day 1. It is important to take your pictures before eating or drinking anything. Choose a time and get used to taking these pictures yourself, as someone may not always be around to help you with this (the same thing for your measurements, do this yourself), this will be known as your before picture.

I usually take pictures from all angles: front, back, both sides, one with a flexed muscle, etc., whichever pictures you decide to take do those same pictures each time you take pictures. This along with how my clothes fit is the tell all of what is really progressing and what is not or still needs work. Once, I have my pictures taken, I then use different apps to create collages to see the progress of the latest picture with the newest picture. I spend hours reviewing every inch of my body on these pictures to make sure I see all my victories. This is the best way to track your weight loss progress.

# Chapter 9: Tricks to Succeed with Intermittent Fasting

## Develop a Schedule for Success

In developing a schedule for your intermittent fasting schedule, you don't want to plan too far into the future. Two weeks at a time is sufficient. The reason for this is that you will be able to plan around upcoming events in order to ensure that you maximize the opportunities available to you. If you wish to plan a month ahead, that is fine, but you need to ensure that you are constantly reassessing your schedule to be certain that you are not caught unaware.

## Slow and Steady Wins the Race

In order to be successful in intermittent fasting, you need to be happy to not have a quick fix. There is no tablet, powder, or liquid that can give you the same benefits that a sustained intermittent fasting lifestyle can, so you have to be willing to work in order to receive those benefits. Any "quick fix" diets, which include you taking any form of medication, are not going to be good for you in the long run. You do not need a tablet to stop you from feeling hungry nor do you need to take any type of drug to help you burn fat. Your body does that very well on its own; you just need to be willing to give it time to remember how.

## Break Your Fast the Right Way

When you break your fast at the beginning of your eating window, you should stick to foods that will not cause your blood sugar to spike. The same goes for your insulin levels, which aren't something that remain consistent when you eat food. It can become impossible to burn fat if there are large amounts of insulin present in your body.

## Fasting Workouts

Fasted workouts have not received much praise due to some findings from studies which claim that working out while you are fasting does not burn more calories than regular training during your eating window or within non-fasting individuals. One of the reasons for this is that most of these results have been flawed due to the fact most of the participants in those studies were given a meal-replacement shake right after their workout, which would have boosted their insulin levels.

## Keep Busy During Fasting Hours

This is a tip that is so close to the truth, to be genuinely successful when fasting: you should keep yourself busy during fasting windows. Keeping yourself busy with work or your favorite pastime or activity may keep your mind off food. Anything, for that matter, that can distract you from thinking of food is best. In doing so, you will allow yourself the opportunity to adapt to fasting as well as help yourself develop that intermittent-fasting mentality that can help drive you to fast for more extended periods.

## Don't make excuses

It is important to not let reasons for not starting an intermittent fast turn into excuses. For example, having a busy schedule or not being able to work in a 12-hour fast are simply reasons that your brain is coming up with to allow you to not try something hard without feeling bad about crying off. The only person who can ensure you are motivated enough to make intermittent fasting work is you, commit to success and follow through on your weight loss goals.

## Find a fasting buddy

It is easier to keep going when you know there is someone else fasting with you. It can be your husband, best friend, or family member. Sit down with them and walk them through the basics of the intermittent fasting technique you have chosen. Use each other as support on those days when one of you doesn't feel like fasting or exercising. It will be more fun when you have someone who you can plan meals with, shop for food with, train with and learn with.

## Set achievable goals

It is best to start with short-term goals that you know you can achieve. Once you attain that goal, reward yourself, but don't do it with junk food. This will help boost your momentum and motivation.

## Keep a progress journal

This is a great way to look at the positive changes you have been experiencing ever since you started your fast. Get a diary and start writing how you feel and all the progress you are making. It is essential to take time to look at how your body and life is transforming. Look at how your clothes fit, the energy you now have to play with your kids, and the way your sleep has improved. Track your positive progress and whip out that journal whenever you feel yourself losing motivation.

## Don't beat yourself up

Yes, there are days when you will fail and succumb to temptation. Things will get rough, and you will grab a cookie and start munching away. Be compassionate with yourself. Don't start talking negatively about yourself just because you didn't do things right.

## Focus On the Good

Throughout the first few weeks, I'm betting that you've found yourself with more energy, especially following the feeding phase, had heightened alertness, euphoria, and even creativity. That felt great, didn't it? You've likely also had more time on your hands recently, particularly so if you are skipping a meal that you usually would spend a bit of time preparing.

## Go slow

These changes take a while, and they do not happen overnight. If you want to lose weight and make sure that it stays at bay, then you'll need to lose weight slowly. You can starve yourself and shed a few pounds, but it will not do you any good. The more gradual and steady your weight loss, the easier it is to maintain. Intermittent fasting is a great dieting option, and it is sustainable. Make sure you go slowly. There is no hurry, and you don't need to jump right in.

## Be Willing to Forgive Yourself

Don't forget, Intermittent Fasting is not a walk in the park. You may realize it's not as easy as people make it out to be. Perhaps you choose to attend a birthday party, and in the process, you ate delicious food instead of sticking to your fasting schedule. That's fine. Just remember, do not beat yourself up about it because this is normal and you're only human. Instead of punishing yourself, realize the mistake, and immediately get back on track and move forward.

## Setbacks are common

Temptation can strike, and there will be times when you might give in to your lures. After all, you are only human. It is okay to face a setback, but don't think of it as a failure. The attitude with which you deal with a delay can set the course for the rest of your diet.

## Be patient

One of the significant obstacles to a diet is the weight loss plateau. You might eat right and exercise correctly, but the numbers on the scales don't seem to change. The scale appears to be stuck for some reason. Well, this is known as the weight-loss plateau, and it is something that every dieter faces. Merely turn around and congratulate yourself for your success so far. It is a part of the process of weight loss.

## Drink plenty of water

While it is easy to see the phrase drink plenty of water and relate it to a command to remain hydrated, what it really means is that while fasting regularly you are going to want to drink a minimum of a gallon of water per day. This practice will not only help you feel full more easily and break your fast early less often, but it will also help your body to continue processing toxins normally during the transition process when it is likely holding on to as much fat as possible.

## Track your progress

Once you begin intermittent fasting, you can start journaling and keeping track of what you are eating. You can easily use your phone as a resource to help you with your intermittent fasting journey. You can use your phone to choose an app that helps with your fasting. A couple of the most popular choices include the Body Fasting app or Fitness Pal. Some apps have extra bonuses you can use, like hiring a personal health coach for extra support.

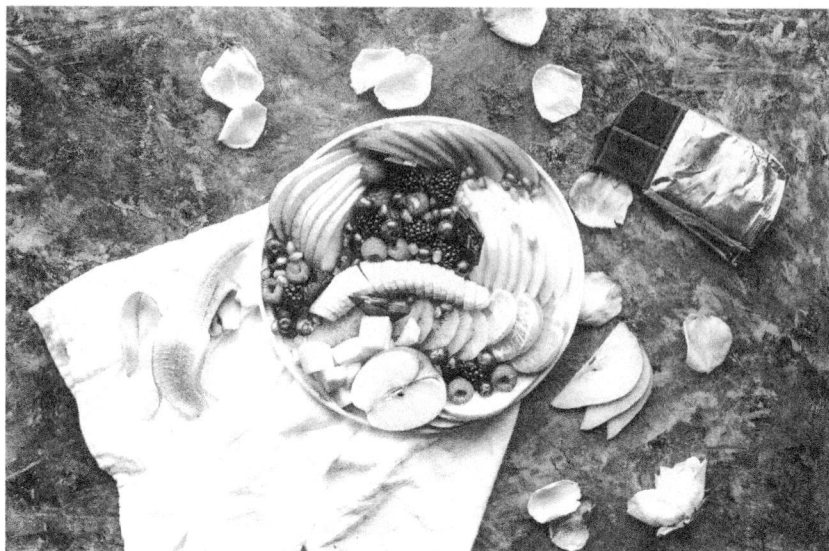

# The best exercises to lose weight after 50 years.

Years Physical activity is the last part of the triad of weight loss, but it is no less important. Exercise pumps blood, releases endorphins after and during workouts, and can help you burn extra calories. The number of calories burned will depend on the type of exercise, duration, and intensity. However, it is generally a small amount and does not approach the number of calories burned by the basal metabolic rate. The average Joe will not have the time or resources to devote significant attention to calorie consumption.

Instead, exercise helps in other ways. In the case of intermittent fasting, it can help regulate energy levels and deplete available glycogen stores, forcing the body to burn fat if it is not already. Do you remember those old-school exercise videos with everyone who talked about "burning"? Exercise will rarely burn fat directly. Fat only burns after glycogen stores are depleted (which takes some time). Most amateur athletes never reach that level of performance.

Sometimes we think that burning some calories (for example, 3,500) is equivalent to burning 1 kg of fat. More specifically, it is burning 3,500 calories, resulting in the loss of a pound of fat, more or less. Many people believe that exercising on an empty stomach is harmful to you. One way this could be true is to cause a significant drop in blood sugar levels. Here, diabetics have to be very careful. The best time to train would be only a few hours after starting a fast when the energy of food is still depleting the body. An exercise of any kind naturally reduces blood sugar levels. If someone cannot regulate their blood sugar levels efficiently (diabetes), they run the risk of having a severe episode of hypoglycemia. Otherwise, the body can detect that blood sugar levels are decreasing and give an adequate response to metabolize glycogen. People who have difficulty training during fasting may choose to "cheat" when they make a small meal before training. Protein shakes are known for this, as they tend to be rich in carbohydrates and proteins. Mixing whey protein with water can vary between 120 and 400 calories, depending on the amount of powder used. Mixing it with milk will significantly increase the caloric content. But you usually don't need protein shakes to exercise.

If you are already used to the fat-burning phase of a low carb diet, it will be easier for you to train regularly, even on an empty stomach. Trying to do a complete workout during the first week of Keto will be difficult. Trying to train in the middle of a fast is also difficult because you will suffer the symptoms of low blood sugar. People with diabetes should take precautions against them. Since a person with diabetes should regularly monitor blood sugar levels, he should schedule a blood meter test just before deciding to exercise. If your blood sugar level is too low, you should not exercise. At a minimum, they should eat something so that these levels return to a healthy interval for physical activity. As with fasting, training should end if symptoms of dizziness, dizziness, vomiting, or loss of consciousness occur.

The types of exercises you decide to perform will depend on your fitness goals. A good general recommendation for people who want to be healthier is resistance training at least twice a week, along with the recommended 150 minutes of moderate to intense aerobic activity. These 150 minutes can be further increased to 300 minutes to receive even more benefits. These include reducing the risk of cardiovascular disease, reducing the risk of cancer, and increasing the weight loss potential of physical activity alone. If a full 300-minute exercise is sustainable per week while fasting will depend on the person's fitness level and the appearance of their fasting routines, for example, someone who is doing the "5: 2" method can only decide No Train in your fast days, others who skip breakfast every day (and fast overnight) may decide to finish training at the end of the fasting period. Breaking the fast with a small meal and then training later is a good option. The exercise becomes a bit more complicated with longer fasts (1-3 days or more). The considerations remain the same, and the risk of hypoglycemia episodes increases.

Benefits of the exercise.

During fasting While exercise on an empty stomach can be expected to present a challenge, there are many benefits. First, exercise without food in the system means that the calories consumed directly affect glycogen stores. In the short term, this means that you will lose weight quickly from the water stored in glycogen and accelerate fat burning. In addition to burning glycogen, you can expect cellular processes to burn at least some fat. They are called AMP kinases and are responsible for accelerating the metabolism of fat in the muscles during workouts. They burn the fat when the body detects that there is enough energy to avoid calories from sugar. The true essence of what happens during quick exercise can get complicated quickly, but your body secretes all kinds of things. Muscles that are exposed to excessive oxidative stress from exercise during fasting become resistant to that stress over time, avoiding the rhythm of the aging process. The brain and muscle tissues go into a rejuvenation process similar to autophagy that keeps things running smoothly. These effects are mainly stimulated during short and intense workouts, such as HIT workouts and resistance training.

Small amounts of human growth hormone (HGH) are released even if you train when glucose stores are low. In turn, this stimulates the secretion of androgens such as testosterone that nourishes the libido and increases lean muscle mass.

Aerobic exercise

Everything that rises and moves is considered aerobic. In particular, it is about increasing your heart rate for prolonged periods. It comes from the word that means "with oxygen," which makes you breathe faster than normal, providing your body with enough oxygen to flow into the blood. Walking, jogging, jumping rope, biking, climbing stairs, and countless sports qualify for aerobic exercise. Current guidelines on physical activity in the United States. UU. Recommend at least 150 minutes.

Of this type of exercise per week. One of the easiest things you can do is walk. Walking is virtually free in most cases and can be a pleasant change of pace. You can bring your dog or friend to accompany you. Fasting aerobic exercise will use glycogen primarily as fuel, depending on how fast it is. If you train immediately after the last meal, you can get an energy boost. Believe it or not, people who exercise in their fasting period report higher energy levels than a non-fast workout. This has to do mainly with HGH body secretion, among other things, to compensate for the lack of readily available energy. But these energy levels are generally reserved for people who are accustomed to fasting. If you try to train during the first weeks of testing, expect great resistance from your body. It is advisable to take things slowly and gradually increase the intensity or duration of fasting workouts. Meanwhile, you can train on days without fasting as usual.

Anaerobic exercise

The opposite of aerobic exercise is the anaerobic type. This covers various forms of resistance training, including bodyweight exercises, strength conditioning, and weightlifting. High-intensity workouts such as HIT and sprint training are also covered. Anaerobic exercise and resistance training, in general, are good for building muscle and strengthening bones. The nervous system also benefits from the mind-body connection used with resistance training. Resistance effectively teaches muscles how to interact with brain signals. Both anaerobic and aerobic exercise should be used together to obtain maximum weight loss results. The main difference between the two is that, under anaerobic conditions, the oxygen that enters the body through the lungs is not enough energy to maintain training. Instead, muscles need to break down sugars (glycogen) to get the energy they need. This decomposition provides weight loss by reducing the amount of glycogen available anytime. Broken glycogen stores become the accumulation of lactic acid; the main reason why muscles feel sore after intense training. The breakdown of muscles also causes a repair mechanism not only to repair torn muscle fibers but also to remove dead components from cells. It would help if you recognized it immediately as autophagy. You will experience an increase in metabolism that lasts hours after training, fasting, or not. Working with fasting, not against you The basic rule for exercising during fasting is not to push things. If dizziness, migraine, vomiting, etc. occur. At any time. While training, it is not a challenge to continue, but a signal that should stop. This is especially true if you train in a warm climate since the temperature will cool your body during overtime.

Hydration is important since dehydration is an important cause of heatstroke. If you plan to lift heavy weights for anaerobic exercise, be sure to exercise lighter than normal on fasting days. Lifting heavy objects with insufficient glycogen stores is a good way to pass out in front of everyone in the gym.

# Chapter 10:     Recipes

## Mango Lime Chia Pudding

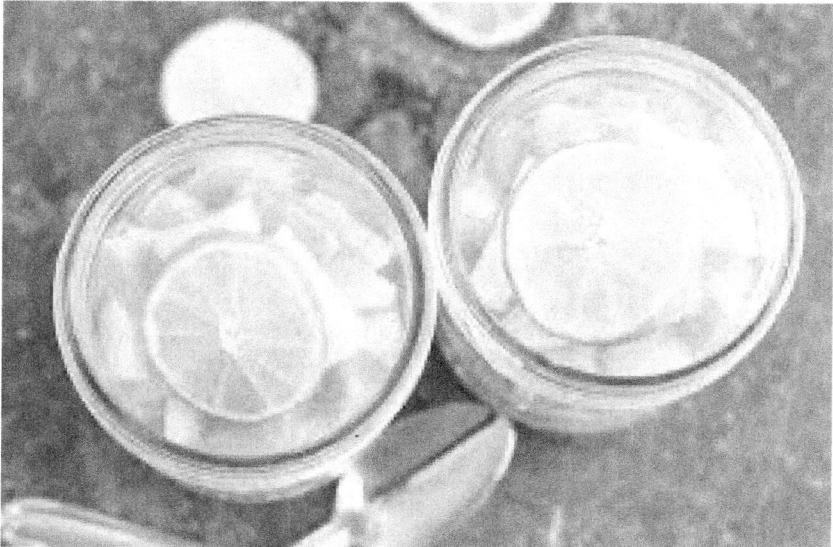

Preparation time: 5 minutes

Cooking time: 30 minutes

Servings: 3

Ingredients:

3 cups fresh or frozen mango chunks

One 15.5-ounce can coconut milk

1 tablespoon lime zest

¼ cup maple syrup

¼ cup freshly squeezed lime juice

¼ cup hemp seeds

1/3 cup chia seeds

Topping options: Approximately 8 cups of any combination of mango, banana, pineapple, or any fruit you'd love with mango and lime. (Banana is a fruit you'd want to wait to add until you are ready to eat the pudding as it browns and gets mushy very quickly once out of its peel)

Directions:

Place mango chunks, coconut milk, lime zest, and maple syrup in a blender. Mix until smooth.

Add hemp and chia seeds in the blender and stir by hand or blend on low to just combine.

This should yield 4 cups of pudding. Portion it as you prefer. One suggestion is to divide into 8 portions, one each in a pint jar, and top with one cup of fresh fruit.

Refrigerate pudding until ready to eat, minimum 4 hours to set. The pudding keeps for 5-7 days.

# Mint Chocolate Truffle Larabar Bites

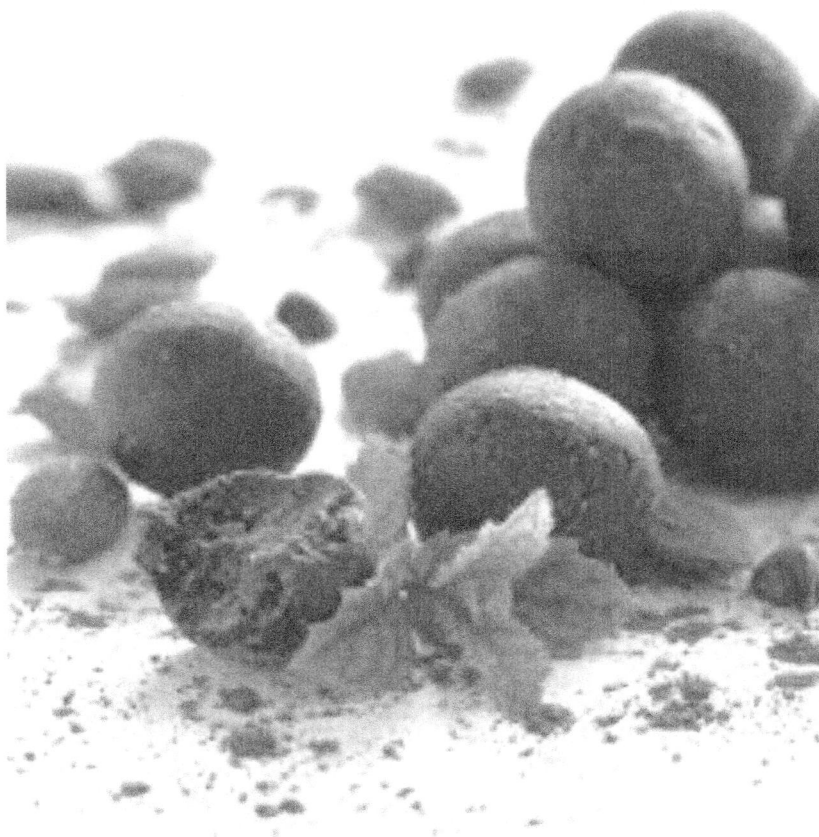

Preparation time: 5 minutes

Cooking time: 45 minutes

Servings: 6

Ingredients:

1 cup vegan chocolate chips (semi-sweet dark chips are

recommended)

10 large Medjool dates

1 ½ cups of raw almonds

¼ cup coconut flour

¼ cup of cocoa powder

¼-1/2 teaspoon peppermint extract

2 tablespoons water

Directions:

Pour almonds into a food processor and chop until a fine flour.

Add chocolate chips, dates, flour and cocoa, and process again until well combined.

Add oil and peppermint extract.

Process one more time until the mix starts balling up.

Taste a small bit and add more peppermint if you wish. Process again if you do.

Remove the blade from the processor and form the dough into balls. Choose whatever size you like, as they do not need to bake and will be good in any portion.

# Keto Chocolate Mousse

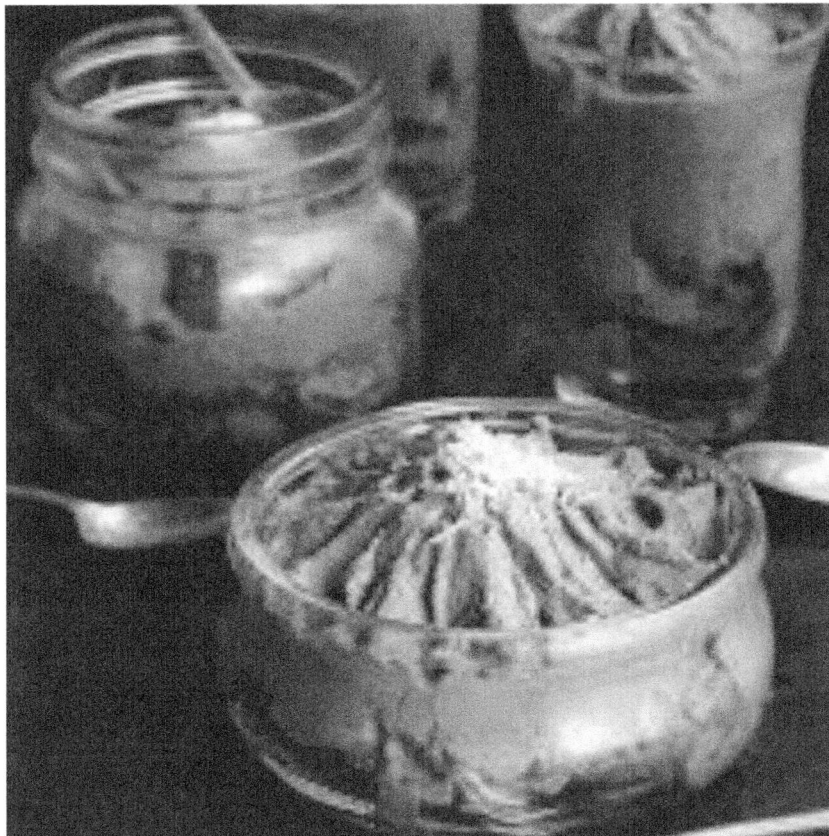

Preparation time: 5 minutes

Cooking time: 40 minutes

Servings: 6

Ingredients:

Cocoa powder – .33 cup

Lakanto monk fruit sweetener – 2 tablespoons

Heavy whipping cream – 1.5 cups

Directions:

Place the heavy cream in a bowl and use a hand mixer or stand mixer to beat it on medium speed.

Once the cream begins to thicken, add the monk fruit sweetener and cocoa and continue to beat it until stiff peaks form.

Serve the mousse immediately or store it in the fridge for up to twenty-four hours before enjoying it. If desired, you can serve it with Lily's stevia-sweetened chocolate for chunks.

# No-Bake Peanut Butter Pie

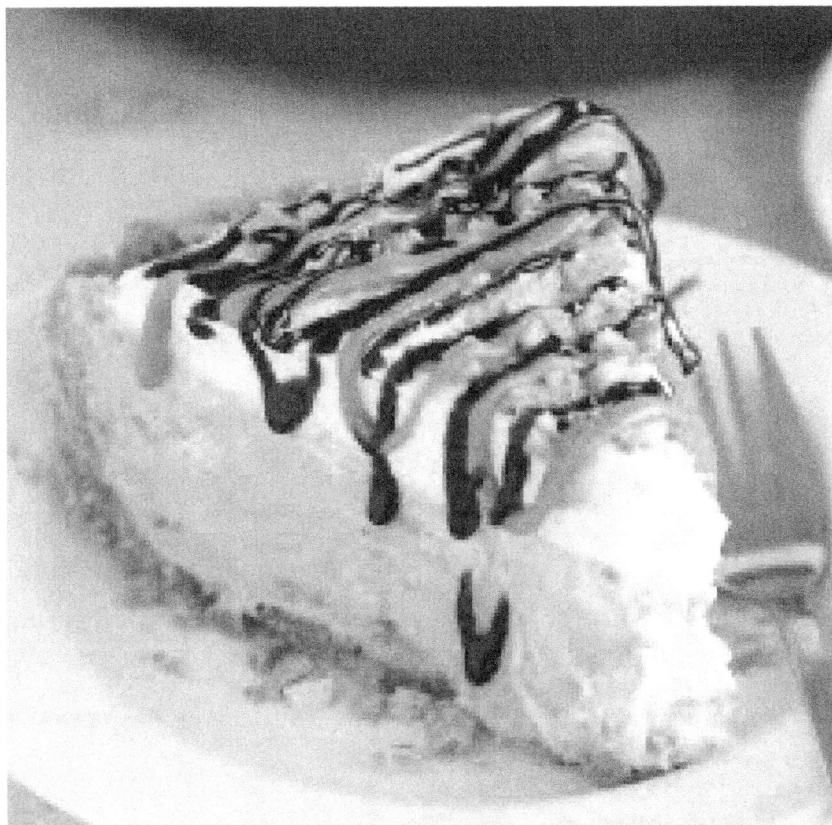

Preparation time: 5 minutes

Cooking time: 60 minutes

Servings: 6

Ingredients:

Almond flour – 1 cup

Butter softened – 2 tablespoons

Vanilla - .5 teaspoon

Lakanto monk fruit sweetener – 1.5 tablespoons

Cocoa powder – 3 tablespoons

Cream cheese softened – 16 ounces

Heavy cream – .75 cup

Vanilla – 2 teaspoons

Swerve confectioner's sweetener - .66 cup

Peanut butter or Sun Butter, unsweetened – .75 cup

Directions:

Combine the almond flour, butter, .5 teaspoon of vanilla, Lakanto sweetener, and cocoa powder in a bowl with a fork until it forms a crumbly mixture. Press this mixture into a nine-inch pie plate and then allow it to chill in the fridge while you prepare the filling.

In a large bowl, beat together the cream cheese, peanut butter, confectioners Swerve, and remaining vanilla until light and creamy. Using a spatula scrape down the sides of the bowl before adding in the heavy cream.

Beat the filling some more until the heavy cream is incorporated and the mixture is once again light and creamy.

Pour the filling into the prepared crust and allow it to chill for two hours before serving. Slice and enjoy.

# Berries with Ricotta Cream

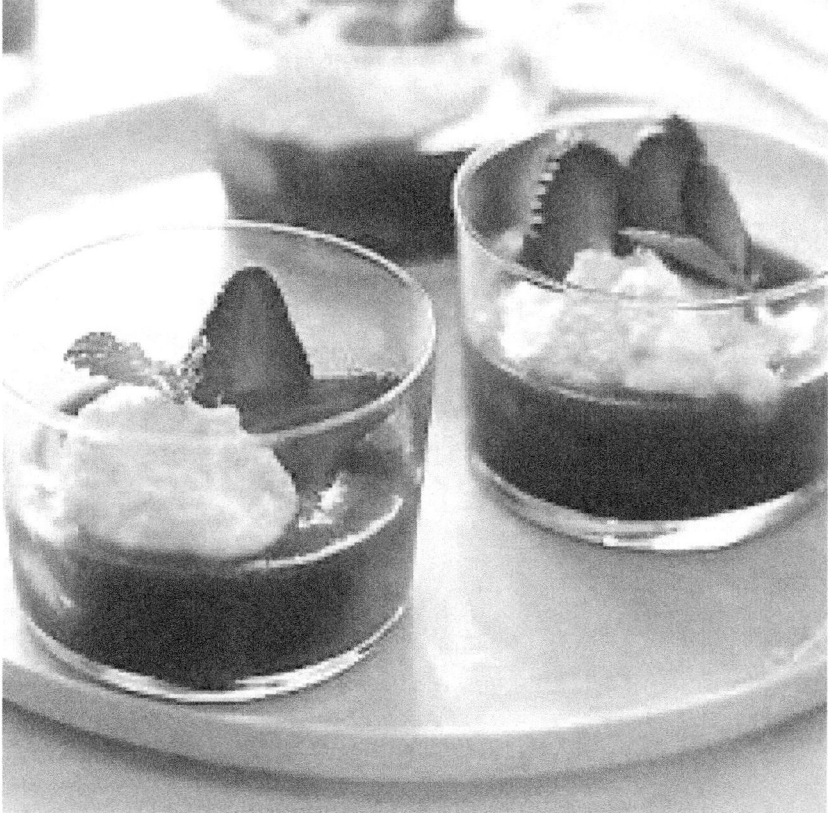

Preparation time: 5 minutes

Cooking time: 40 minutes

Servings: 6

Ingredients:

Ricotta, whole milk – 1.5 cups

Heavy cream – 2 tablespoons

Lemon zest – 1.5 teaspoons

Swerve confectioner's sweetener – .25 cup

Vanilla extract – 1 teaspoon

Blackberries - .5 cup

Raspberries - .5 cup

Blueberries - .5 cup

Directions:

In a large bowl, add all of the ingredients, except for the berries, and whip them together with a hand mixer until completely smooth.

Set out four parfait glasses and divide half of the berries between all of them. Top the berries with half of the ricotta mixture, the remaining half of the berries, and lastly, the second half of the ricotta mixture.

Serve the parfaits immediately or within the next twenty-four hours.

# Easy Chocolate Pudding

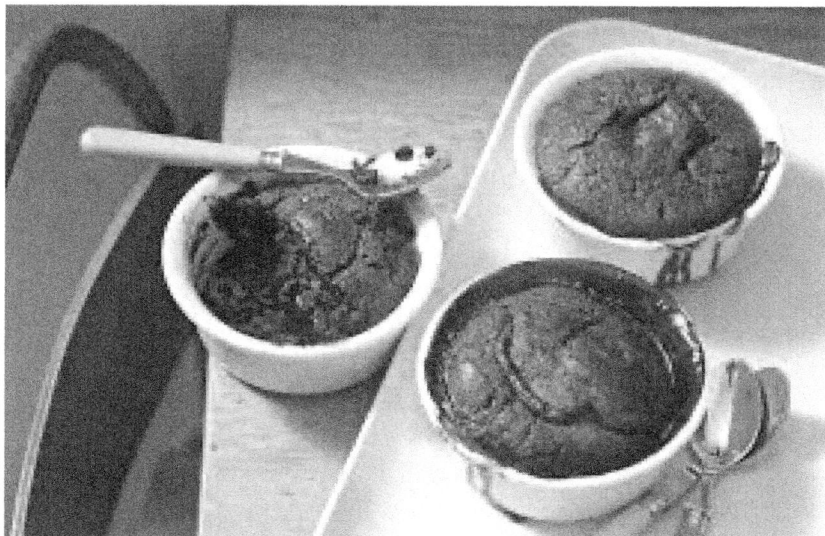

Preparation time: 5 minutes

Cooking time: 30 minutes

Servings: 6

Ingredients:

1 ½ cups organic coconut cream from a can

½ cup raw cacao powder (sifted unsweetened cocoa powder works as well)

6 tablespoons pure maple syrup (may adjust to up to 8 tablespoons, depending on how sweet you like it)

2 teaspoons pure vanilla extract

Fine-grain sea salt

Directions:

In a small saucepan over low heat, whisk coconut cream, cacao, and maple syrup until smooth. A smaller whisk my make a smoother mixture. Continue to cook over low/medium for 2 minutes, or until the mixture just starts to come to a boil with small bubbles.

Remove from heat. Add salt and vanilla. Stir. Taste and add more maple if you'd like a sweeter pudding.

Pour into individual containers/bowls or keep in one larger bowl to set.

Cover and refrigerate until set, or overnight for a thick and creamy pudding. Makes 4 servings.

# Pan-fried Jackfruit over Pasta with Lemon Coconut Cream Sauce

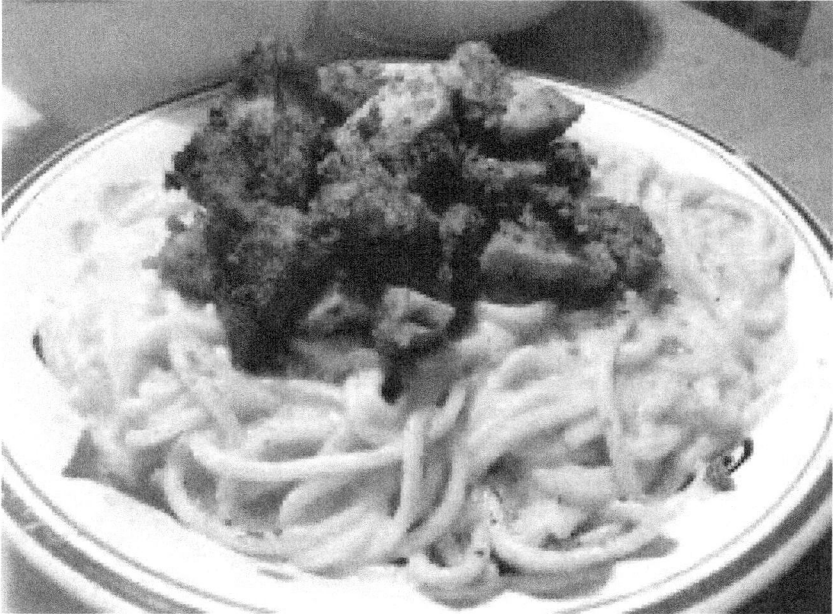

Preparation time: 5 minutes

Cooking time: 30 minutes

Servings: 6

Ingredients:

1 lb. pasta of choice

2 cans jackfruit in brine

2 tablespoons flour of choice

Garlic powder, dried oregano, paprika, black pepper, kosher salt to taste

2 tablespoons vegetable oil

4 tablespoons vegan butter

2 cups of coconut milk

Juice of 1 lemon

2 tablespoons grated vegan parmesan cheese

1 pinch ground nutmeg

1 teaspoon lemon zest (can use the same lemon from juice)

Fresh basil leaves, chopped for garnish

Directions:

Cook pasta until al dente. Drain the pasta but reserve 1 cup of the pasta water. Set it aside for now.

While the pasta is cooking, drain the jackfruit and cut each piece in half. Pat jackfruit dry.

Mix flour with garlic powder, oregano, paprika, pepper, and salt in a separate bowl.

Toss flour mixture with jackfruit.

Heat vegetable oil in a skillet. Pan-fry the jackfruit until crisp on both sides. It takes around ten minutes in total.

Transfer the jackfruit to a plate lined with a paper towel and set aside.

In a large saucepan or skillet, melt vegan butter. Add coconut milk and lemon juice. Then add parmesan cheese and nutmeg. Cook until sauce is thick.

Add cooked pasta and half of the reserved pasta water to skillet. Toss to coat all pasta.

Cook until everything is hot and the sauce is to desired consistency and pasta is heated through. If the sauce is too thick, continue to use remaining pasta water.

Turn off heat. Add lemon zest and add pepper and salt to taste. Sprinkle parmesan and basil leaves. Add pan-fried jackfruit on top when serving.

# Butternut Squash Tacos with Tempeh Chorizo

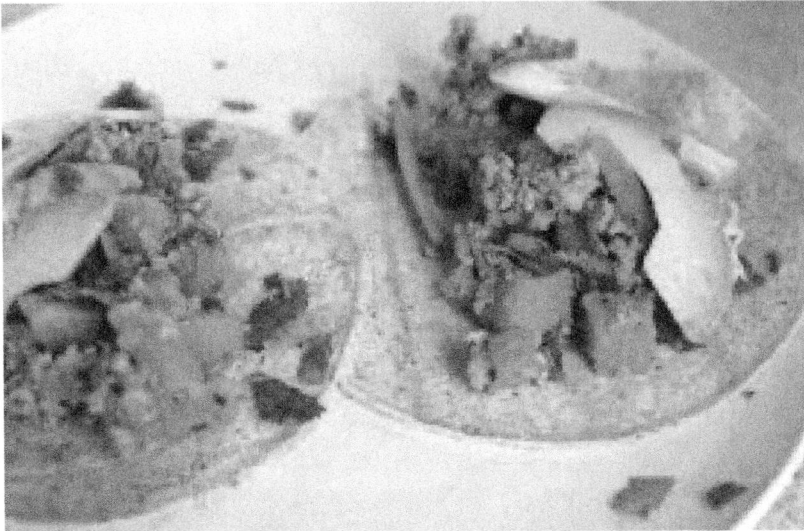

Preparation time: 5 minutes

Cooking time: 50 minutes

Servings: 5

Ingredients:

One 8-ounce package tempeh

½ cup of filtered water

¼ cup apple cider vinegar

2 cups butternut squash, peeled, cut into cubes

1 teaspoon chili powder

½ teaspoon smoked paprika

½ teaspoon cumin

½ teaspoon garlic powder

½ teaspoon oregano

A dash of cayenne

1 tablespoon nutritional yeast

A few dashes of liquid smoke

Black pepper and sea salt to taste

½ cup thinly julienned carrot (optional)

8 corn tortillas (or whatever you have on hand)

1 large avocado, pitted and sliced

Cilantro, chopped

Instructions:

Cut the tempeh into two parts. Steam for 10 min. Place in a large bowl and tear apart into small pieces either with your hands (after it's cooled) or with a pastry cutter.

While tempeh is steaming, bring water and vinegar to a boil in a small skillet.

Add spices, squash, liquid smoke, nutritional yeast, and a pinch of sea salt to skillet. Coat well and simmer covered, stirring occasionally. Add carrots and tempeh, covering again. Simmer a little while longer, stirring to prevent sticking. Uncover and season with pepper and salt.

Fill warmed tortillas with squash and tempeh mix and top with avocado and cilantro.

# Coated Cauliflower Head

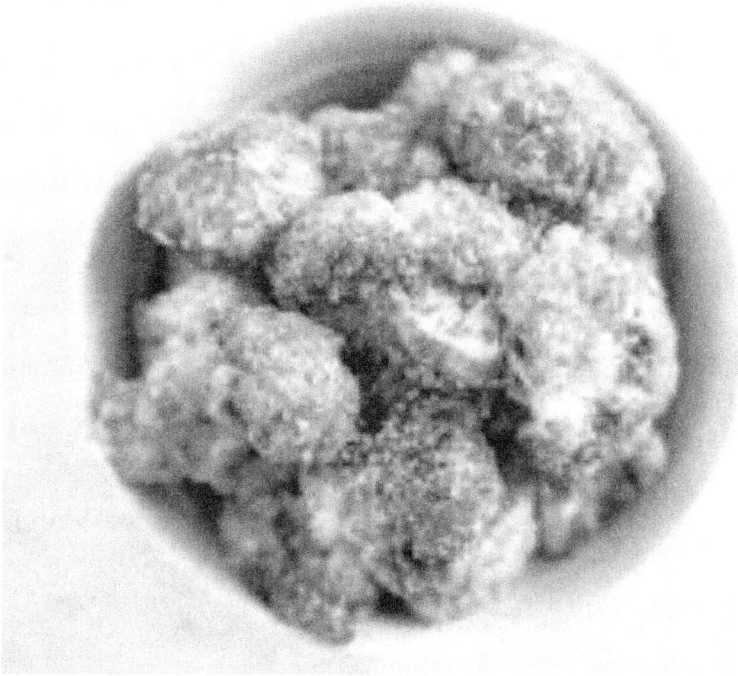

Preparation time: 10 minutes

Cooking time: 40 minutes

Servings: 6

Ingredients:

2-pound cauliflower head

3 tablespoons olive oil

1 tablespoon butter, softened

1 teaspoon ground coriander

1 teaspoon salt

1 egg, whisked

1 teaspoon dried cilantro

1 teaspoon dried oregano

1 teaspoon tahini paste

Directions:

Trim cauliflower head if needed.

Preheat oven to 350F.

In the mixing bowl, mix up together olive oil, softened butter, ground coriander, salt, whisked egg, dried cilantro, dried oregano, and tahini paste.

Then brush the cauliflower head with this mixture generously and transfer in the tray.

Bake the cauliflower head for 40 minutes.

Brush it with the remaining oil mixture every 10 minutes.

# Artichoke Petals Bites

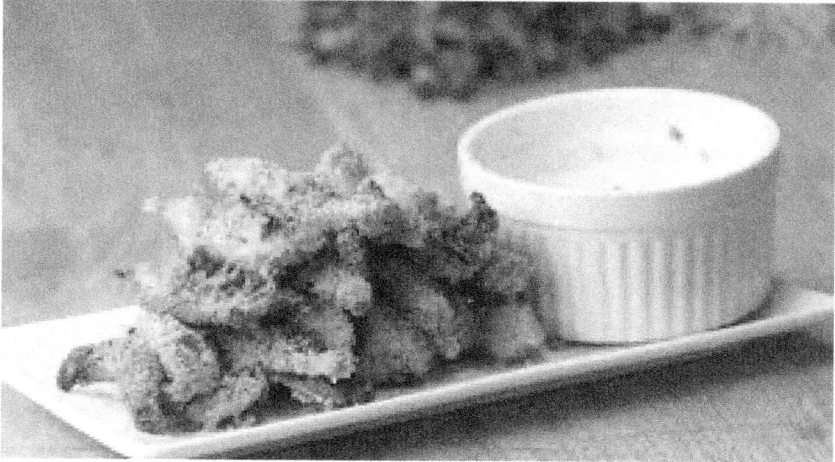

Preparation time: 10 minutes

Cooking time: 10 minutes

Servings: 8

Directions:

8 oz. artichoke petals, boiled, drained, without salt

½ cup almond flour

4 oz. Parmesan, grated

2 tablespoons almond butter, melted

Instructions:

In the mixing bowl, mix up together almond flour and grated Parmesan.

Preheat the oven to 355F.

Dip the artichoke petals in the almond butter and then coat in the almond flour mixture.

Place them in the tray.

Transfer the tray in the preheated oven and cook the petals for 10 minutes.

Chill the cooked petal bites little before serving.

# Stuffed Beef Loin in Sticky Sauce

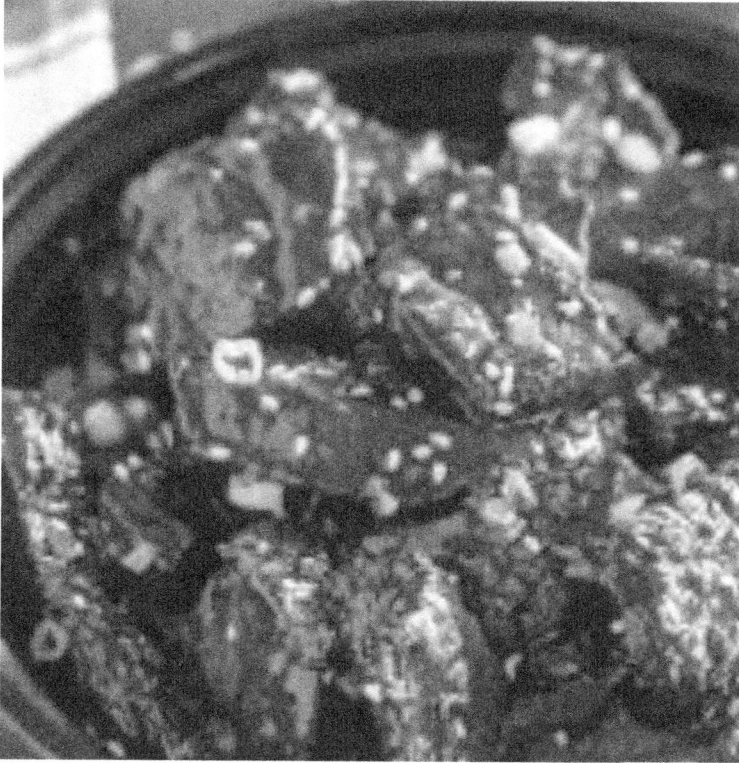

Preparation time: 15 minutes

Cooking time: 6 minutes

Servings: 4

Ingredients:

1 tablespoon Erythritol

1 tablespoon lemon juice

4 tablespoons water

1 tablespoon butter

½ teaspoon tomato sauce

¼ teaspoon dried rosemary

9 oz. beef loin

3 oz. celery root, grated

3 oz. bacon, sliced

1 tablespoon walnuts, chopped

¾ teaspoon garlic, diced

2 teaspoons butter

1 tablespoon olive oil

1 teaspoon salt

½ cup of water

Directions:

Cut the beef loin into the layer and spread it with the dried rosemary, butter, and salt.

Then place over the beef loin: grated celery root, sliced bacon, walnuts, and diced garlic.

Roll the beef loin and brush it with olive oil.

Secure the meat with the help of the toothpicks.

Place it in the tray and add a ½ cup of water.

Cook the meat in the preheated to 365F oven for 40 minutes.

Meanwhile, make the sticky sauce: mix up together Erythritol, lemon juice, 4 tablespoons of water, and butter.

Preheat the mixture until it starts to boil.

Then add tomato sauce and whisk it well.

Bring the sauce to boil and remove from the heat.

When the beef loin is cooked, remove it from the oven and brush with the cooked sticky sauce very generously.

Slice the beef roll and sprinkle with the remaining sauce.

# Vegan Fish Sticks and Tartar Sauce

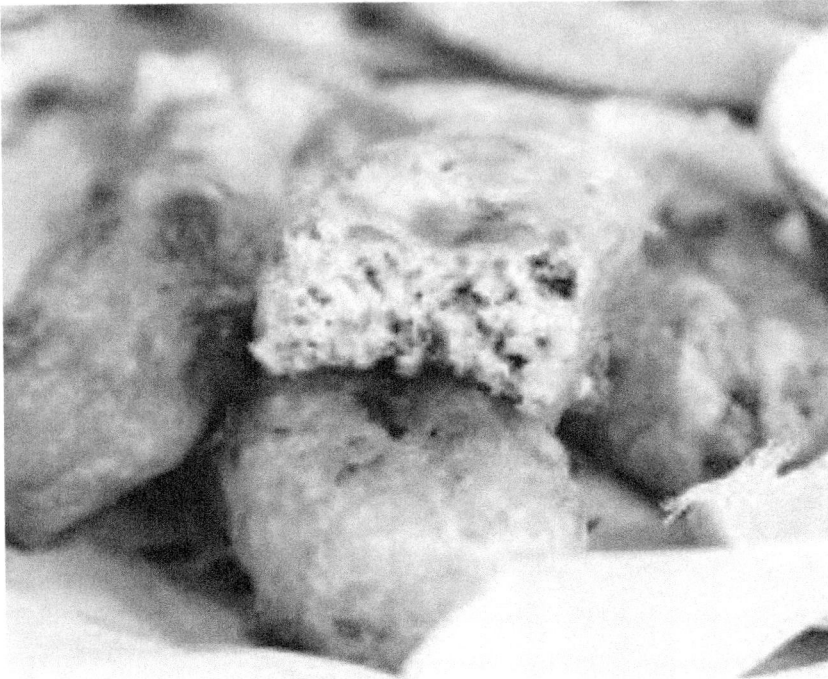

Preparation time: 5 minutes

Cooking time: 80 minutes

Servings: 6

Ingredients:

Fish Sticks:

12-ounce package extra-firm tofu

½ cup cornmeal

1 tablespoon garlic powder

1 tablespoon dried basil

2 tablespoons dulse flakes

1 tablespoon onion powder

½ cup whole wheat flour (rice flour is a good gluten-free option)

10 turns fresh black pepper

1 tablespoon of sea salt

¼ cup non-dairy milk, unsweetened

1 cup high-heat oil for frying

Vegan Tartar Sauce:

¼ cup sweet pickle relish

½ cup vegan mayo

½ teaspoon sugar

½ teaspoon lemon juice

5 turns fresh black pepper

Directions:

Rinse tofu and drain in a colander. Placing a heavy plate on tofu with a heavy item on top will help drain better. Set it aside.

In a medium bowl, mix the flour, cornmeal, garlic powder, basil, onion powder, dulse flakes, pepper, and salt. Whisk together. Set the mix aside.

Set tofu on cutting board. Cut into quarters.

Slice tofu into thin pieces. You should have 28-32 pieces in total.

In a large cast-iron skillet, heat oil on medium/low heat.

In a small bowl, pour non-dairy milk.

Dip each piece of tofu in non-dairy milk. Immediately dip in breading, coating all sides evenly. Repeat until all pieces are coated.

The oil will start to splatter when hot enough. At that point, add tofu pieces to skillet. Repeat until all pieces are cooked.

Each side will cook for about 2-3 minutes. Watch for golden brown color. Place tofu pieces on a brown paper bag as you remove them from pan to soak up excess oil.

Repeat as necessary until all tofu is cooked. Cool before serving. Mix all tartar sauce ingredients until an even and creamy sauce is made. Enjoy!

# Vegan Philly Cheesesteak

Preparation time: 5 minutes

Cooking time: 40 minutes

Servings: 4

Ingredients:

6-8 sliced Portobello mushrooms

4 cloves garlic, minced

1 tablespoon olive oil

1 whole clove garlic

½ teaspoon black pepper

1 teaspoon dried thyme

½ large diced onion

A dash of kosher salt

1 tablespoon vegan Worcestershire sauce

Hoagie rolls or another small loaf of bread of choice

1 cup shredded vegan cheddar cheese

Vegan mayo (optional)

Directions:

Preheat the broiler.

In a deep skillet, heat olive oil. Brown mushrooms in oil, about 10 min.

Add thyme, garlic, and pepper until evenly coated.

Add onion and salt. Mushrooms must be well cooked before adding salt. Cook until onion is caramelized and softened, which should be for about 5 minutes. Add Worcestershire sauce and mix well.

Slice the bread lengthwise. Coat open sides of bread with olive oil or cooking spray. To add garlic flavor, cut the whole garlic clove, cut off the tip, and put on the oiled side of bread. Garlic powder is also a good substitute.

If desired, add optional vegan mayo. Place bread on cookie sheet. Fill loaves with mushrooms and top with shredded vegan cheddar cheese.

# Basil and Cherry Tomato Breakfast

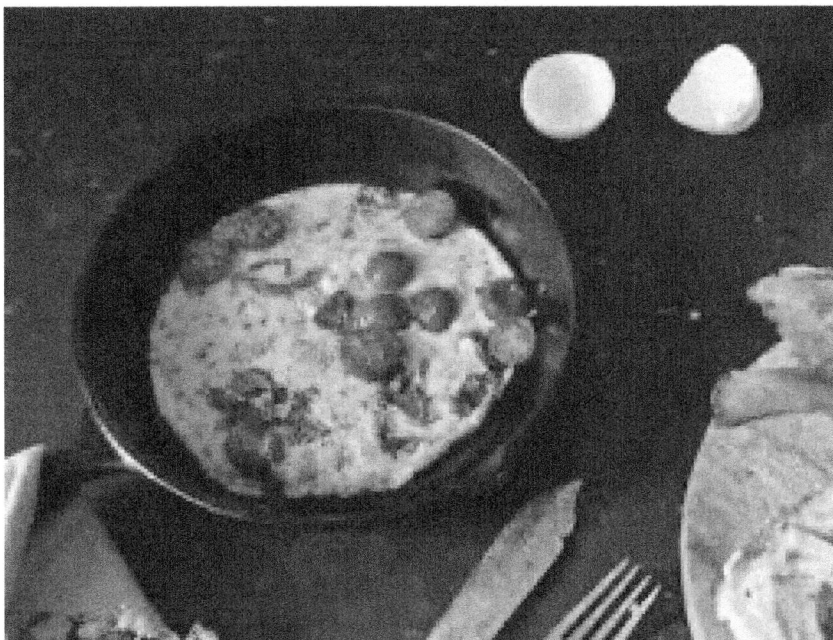

Preparation time: 4 minutes

Cooking time: 4 hours

Servings: 4

Ingredients:

1 tablespoon olive oil

2 yellow onions, chopped

2 pounds cherry tomatoes, halved

3 tablespoons tomato puree

2 garlic cloves, minced

A pinch of sea salt and black pepper

1 bunch basil, chopped

Directions:

Grease the slow cooker with the oil, add all the ingredients, cover and cook on high for 4 hours.

Stir the mixture, divide it into bowls and serve for breakfast.

# Carrot Breakfast Salad

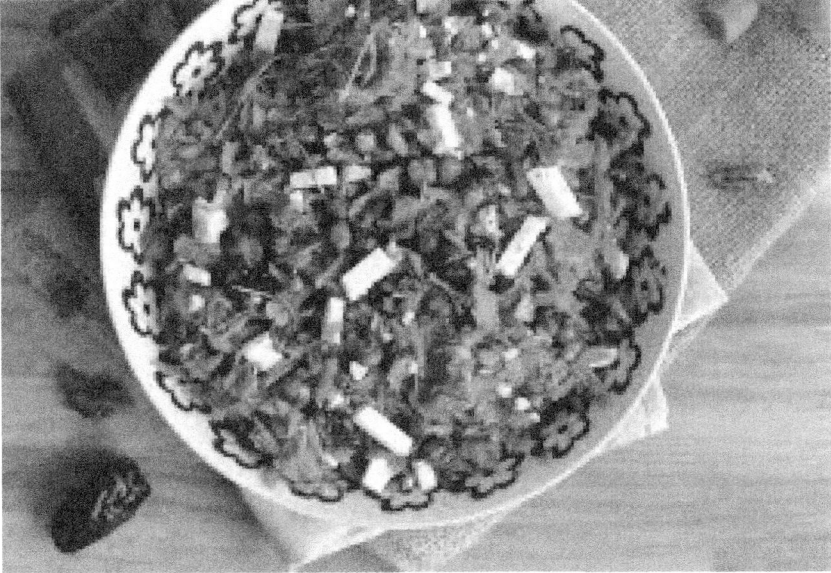

Preparation time: 5 minutes

Cooking time: 4 hours

Servings: 4

Ingredients:

2 tablespoons olive oil

2 pounds baby carrots, peeled and halved

3 garlic cloves, minced

2 yellow onions, chopped

½ cup vegetable stock

1/3 cup tomatoes, crushed

A pinch of salt and black pepper

Directions:

In your slow cooker, combine all the ingredients, cover and cook on high for 4 hours.

Divide into bowls and serve for breakfast.

Place in broiler until cheese has melted, which should be 4-5 minutes.

# Greek Breakfast Covers

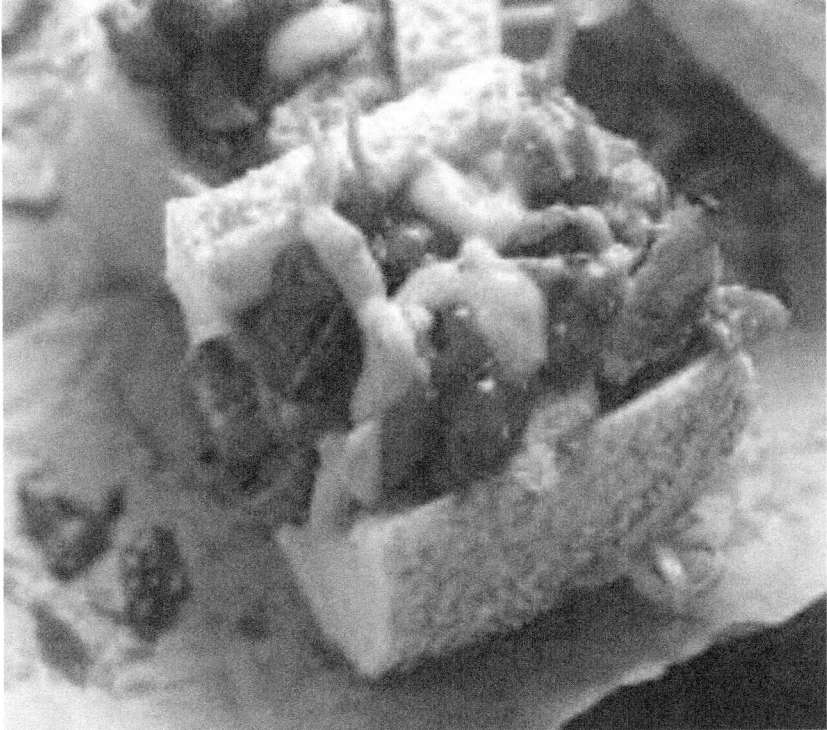

Preparation time: 10 minutes

Cooking time: 5 minutes

Servings: 2

This recipe is simply as satisfying as that fast-food breakfast sandwich. However, this wrap has far less fat and fewer calories. It's a fast breakfast to make ahead of time and reheat in the early morning or when you get to work.

Ingredients

1 teaspoon olive oil.

1/2 cup fresh baby spinach leaves.

1 tablespoon fresh basil.

4 egg whites, beaten.

1/2 teaspoon salt.

1/4 teaspoon newly ground black pepper.

1/4 cup crumbled low-fat feta cheese.

2 (8-inch) whole-wheat tortillas.

Directions:

In a little skillet, heat the olive oil over medium heat. Add the spinach and basil to the pan and sauté for about 2 minutes, or simply up until the spinach is wilted.

Include the egg whites to the pan, season with the salt and pepper, and sauté stirring typically, for about 2 minutes more, or up until the egg whites are firm.

Remove it from the heat and sprinkle with the feta cheese.

Heat the tortillas in the microwave for 20 to 30 seconds, or just up until softened and warm. Divide the eggs between the tortillas and finish up burrito-style.

# Avocado and Fennel Salad with Balsamic Vinaigrette

Preparation time: 15 minutes

Cooking time: 0 minute

Servings: 2

This salad contains a wonderful mix of tasty citrus, smooth avocado, and anise-flavored fennel. Tossed with a fast and straightforward balsamic vinaigrette, it's the best lunch or light dinner for warm days.

 Ingredients

1 tablespoon light olive oil.

1 tablespoon balsamic vinegar.

1/4 teaspoon salt.

1/2 cup fennel, sliced.

1/2 avocado, diced.

1/2 cup mandarin oranges, drained.

1 cup sliced romaine lettuce.

1/4 teaspoon freshly ground black pepper.

Directions:

In a medium blending bowl, integrate the olive oil, balsamic vinegar, salt, and pepper, and whisk till well combined and a little thickened. This is your balsamic vinaigrette.

Include the fennel, avocado, oranges, and lettuce; toss until the veggies are well covered with a dressing. Divide between 2 salad plates and serve cold.

# Penne Pasta with Vegetables

Preparation time: 15 minutes

Cooking time: 15 minutes

Servings: 2

Even on fasting days, you can delight in a light pasta meal. This one is chock-full of vitamin C and iron from the spinach and tomatoes and provides lots of flavor and satisfaction

Ingredients

1 teaspoon salt, divided.

3/4 cup raw penne pasta.

1 tablespoon olive oil.

1 tablespoon chopped garlic.

1 teaspoon chopped fresh oregano.

1 cup sliced fresh mushrooms.

10 cherry tomatoes, cut in half.

1 cup fresh spinach leaves.

1/2 teaspoon freshly ground black pepper.

1 tablespoon shredded Parmesan cheese.

Directions:

In a big pan, pour 1quart water to a boil.

Include 1/2 teaspoon of the salt and the penne, and cook according to package directions, or until (about 9 minutes).

Drain but do not wash the penne, scheduling about 1/4 cup pasta water.

Meanwhile, in a big frying pan, heat the olive oil over medium-high heat. Include the garlic, oregano, and mushrooms, and sauté for 4 to 5 minutes, or till the mushrooms are golden.

Add the tomatoes and spinach, season with the remaining 1/2 teaspoon salt and the black pepper, and sauté for 3 to 4 minutes, or up until the spinach is wilted.

Add the drained pipes pasta to the skillet, together with 2 to 3 tablespoons of the pasta water.

Cook, constantly stirring, for 2 to 3 minutes, or until the pasta is glowing and the water has actually cooked off.

Divide the pasta in between 2 shallow bowls and sprinkle with the Parmesan cheese. Serve hot or at space temperature level.

# Hearty Shrimp and Kale Soup

Preparation time: 15 minutes

Cooking time: 35 minutes

Servings: 2

This delicious soup loads many anti-oxidants from the carrots and kale, plus a healthy amount of protein from the shrimp and beans. It's delicious, basic, and pleasing.

Ingredients

1 teaspoon olive oil.

2 cloves garlic.

1/4 cup chopped onion.

2 cups sliced fresh kale.

1 cup thinly sliced fresh carrots.

1/2 teaspoon salt.

1 1/2 cups vegetable stock.

8 medium (36-- 40 counts) raw shrimp, peeled and halved.

1 cup canned fantastic northern beans drained pipes.

1/4 cup sliced fresh parsley.

1/4 teaspoon freshly ground black pepper.

Directions:

In a medium saucepan, heat the olive oil over medium heat.

Add the garlic onion, kale, and carrots, and sauté for 5 minutes, stirring frequently.

Season the veggies with the salt and pepper, then add the veggie stock.

Simmer, uncovered, for 30 minutes, or until the carrots are fork-tender.

Increase the heat to high and bring the soup to a boil. Add the shrimp and cook for 2 minutes, or until the shrimp are pink and somewhat company. Minimize the heat to low.

Use a fork to mash about one-quarter of the beans. Stir all the beans into the soup and add the parsley. Simmer for 2 minutes, or until heated up through.

Ladle into soup bowls and serve hot.

# Pork Loin Chops with Mango Salsa

Preparation time: 10 minutes

Cooking time: 10 minutes

Servings: 2

This dish is bursting with taste and is pleasing enough to make you forget that you are fasting. The salsa is even much better prepared a day ahead, so allow it to marinate in the fridge overnight with the pork chops.

Ingredients

2 pork loin chops, 3/4 inch thick.

1/2 cup lime juice.

Juice of 1 big orange.

1 large simply ripe mango, peeled and diced.

1/2 cup diced green bell pepper.

1/2 cup diced red bell pepper.

1 small jalapeño pepper, seeded and diced.

1 tablespoon sliced fresh cilantro.

1/2 cup diced red onion - 1 tablespoon chopped fresh parsley.

1/2 teaspoon salt.

1/4 teaspoon newly ground black pepper.

Directions:

Place the pork chops in a freezer bag and include the lime and orange juices. Seal, shake to mix well and place in the refrigerator overnight.

In a little bowl, combine the mango, red onion, bell peppers, jalapeño, cilantro, and parsley. Stir to integrate effectively.

Cover and refrigerate overnight.

Preheat the grill and line a baking pan with aluminum foil.

Season each pork slice on both sides with the salt and pepper. Put on the pan and broil for 4 to 5 minutes on one side, then turn over and broil for 4 to 5 minutes more.

Place each pork slice on a plate, spoon the salsa over the top, and serve.

# Nutty Peach Parfaits.

Preparation time: 15 minutes

Cooking time: 0 minute

Servings: 4

These parfaits may look quite, but they're even healthier than they look. The walnuts include omega-3 fats and fiber as well as crunch, and the Greek yogurt has as much as fourteen grams of protein per cup.

Ingredients

4 medium peaches, sliced.

4 (6-ounce) containers vanilla Greek yogurt.

1/2 cup unsalted walnuts, chopped.

Directions:

Divide the ingredients in between 4 parfait or dessert dishes. Start with a layer of peaches; then include a spoonful of yogurt and after that, scatter the walnuts.

# Salmon and Tomato Egg Sandwiches.

Preparation time: 15 minutes

Cooking time: 5 minutes

Servings: 4

This breakfast sandwich is far healthier and more considerable than anything you can get at the drive-through; it's likewise a lot tastier, but only takes a few minutes to prepare.

Ingredients

4 light multigrain English muffins.

1 teaspoon olive oil.

6 ounces canned pink salmon.

1 cup diced tomatoes.

8 large eggs, beaten.

1/2 teaspoon salt.

1/4 teaspoon freshly ground black pepper.

1 cup fresh arugula.

Directions:

Toast the English muffins while you prepare the eggs.

In a medium skillet, heat the olive oil over medium-high heat. Include the salmon and tomatoes to the pan, and sauté, stirring regularly, for 4 minutes.

Pour the eggs over the top, season with the salt and pepper, and scramble.

stirring often, for about 2 minutes, or up until the eggs are set.

Place the English muffin halves on 4 plates and leading each bottom half with.

one-quarter of the egg mixture. Leading with arugula and the other muffin half.

# Cocoa-Banana Breakfast Smoothie

Preparation time: 15 minutes

Cooking time: 0 minute

Servings: 4

This healthy smoothie takes simply seconds to make, but it's packed with nutrition. The Greek yogurt provides a healthy dosage of protein and the bananas are a fantastic source of potassium.

Ingredients

24 ounces vanilla Greek yogurt

2 medium bananas, cut into pieces

1 teaspoon honey

2 tablespoons unsweetened cocoa powder

1/2 cup low-fat milk

1/2 cup ice cubes

Directions:

Place the yogurt and bananas into a blender and blend on high until the bananas are smooth. Add the honey, milk, and cocoa and blend again till well incorporated.

Include the ice and mix again, pulsing as required, till the mix is smooth and thick.

# Cranberry-Walnut Whole Wheat Pancakes

Preparation time:

Cooking time:

Servings: 4

These pancakes are a delicious method to start your day. The cranberries are tart yet sweet, and the walnuts add crunch and texture to this convenience classic.

Ingredients

1/2 cup fresh cranberries

3/4 cup whole wheat flour

2 tablespoons sugar

1 tablespoon baking powder

1/4 teaspoon salt

1/2 teaspoon ground nutmeg

1/2 teaspoon pure vanilla extract

1 1/4 cup low-fat milk

1 big egg, beaten

1/2 cup chopped walnuts

1 tablespoon coconut oil, divided

Directions:

In a little bowl, combine the cranberries with a handful of the entire wheat flour, tossing them well to coat.

In a large mixing bowl, integrate the staying flour, sugar, baking powder, salt, and nutmeg, stirring to blend well.

Add the egg, vanilla, and milk and stir to mix, however do not overmix. The batter ought to remain somewhat lumpy. Carefully fold in the cranberries and walnuts

(with flour) and set the batter aside for 10 minutes.

In a large heavy frying pan, heat about 1/2 teaspoon of the coconut oil over medium heat. Ladle enough batter into the pan to make a 6-inch pancake

Cook for about 2 minutes, or till the edges are bubbly, then turn the pancake and prepare for 1 minute more. Transfer to a plate and cover to keep warm while you make the remainder of the pancakes. Include extra coconut oil to the pan as needed.

To serve, location 2 pancakes on each plate and top with warm maple syrup, honey, or molasses.

# Scrambled Egg Soft Tacos

Preparation time: 10 minutes

Cooking time: 5 minutes

Servings: 4

Finding alternatives to junk food for your early morning meal can be a challenge, however, this dish is an outstanding one to try. It's filled with southwestern flavor, however low in both fat and calories.

Ingredients

8 (6-inch) entire wheat tortillas

1 teaspoon olive oil

2 green onions, chopped

1/2 teaspoon cayenne pepper

12 big eggs, beaten

1 cup moderate chunky salsa

1 cup low-fat shredded cheddar cheese

Directions

Place the tortillas on a plate, top with a moist paper towel, and microwave for 30 to 45 seconds, or just up until pliable and warm. Cover with a second plate or pot cover to keep warm.

In a large heavy skillet, heat the olive oil over medium heat. Add the green onions and sauté for 1 minute. Stir the cayenne into the eggs, then put them into the skillet. Scramble, stirring continuously, up until the eggs are prepared, about 5 minutes.

Divide the egg mix uniformly in between the tortillas, leading the tortillas with 2 tablespoons each salsa and cheddar cheese, and fold the tacos in half.

# Herb and Swiss Frittata

Preparation time: 30 minutes

Cooking time: 22 minutes

This frittata looks like something you 'd see in a dining establishment, however it takes just a couple of minutes to prepare. You'll enjoy the layered tastes, courtesy of moderate Swiss cheese and fresh herbs.

Servings: 4

Ingredients

2 teaspoons olive oil

8 large eggs, beaten

1/2 teaspoon salt

1/2 teaspoon freshly ground black pepper

2 teaspoons chopped fresh parsley

2 teaspoons chopped fresh marjoram

1 teaspoon chopped fresh basil

1/2 cup shredded low-fat Swiss cheese

Directions:

Pre-heat the oven to 375 degrees F.

Heat the olive oil in a large ovenproof skillet over high heat. Put in the eggs, dispersing them equally around the skillet. Season with the salt and pepper.

Remove the skillet from the heat and spray the marjoram, basil, and parsley evenly over the top of the eggs. Leading with the Swiss cheese.

Location the skillet in the middle of the oven and bake for 18 to 22 minutes, or until a toothpick inserted into the center comes out clean.

To serve, cut into four wedges and serve hot.

# Vanilla-Almond Protein Shake

Preparation time: 10 minutes

Cooking time: 0 minute

Servings: 4

This breakfast shake has plenty of protein and healthy fats to keep you going on even your toughest mornings. This is a great method to get your breakfast to go—simply put into a travel mug and drink on your method.

Ingredients

2 cups cold water.

4 scoops unflavored whey protein.

isolate powder - 1/4 cup almond.

butter.

2 tablespoons honey.

1/2 teaspoon almond extract.

1/2 teaspoon ground nutmeg.

10 ice cubes.

Directions:

In a mixer, integrate the cold water, protein powder, almond butter, honey, almond extract, and nutmeg. Mix on high for about 30 seconds, or till smooth.

Add the ice cubes and blend once again until thick and creamy. Consume right away.

# Scrambled Eggs with Mushrooms and Onions

Preparation time: 10 minutes

Cooking time: 5 minute

Servings: 4

These eggs are cook up in a hurry however has a taste that will plead you to decrease and enjoy it. This makes a great sandwich filling, too. , if you must consume breakfast on the run, a whole-wheat pita pocket is an excellent option.

Ingredients

1 teaspoon olive oil.

1 cup sliced fresh mushrooms.

1/4 cup thinly sliced yellow onion.

1 tablespoon sliced fresh.

tarragon.

1/2 cup chopped fresh parsley.

1/2 teaspoon salt.

1/2 teaspoon newly ground black pepper.

8 big eggs, beaten.

Directions:

In a large heavy frying pan, heat the olive oil over medium heat. Add the mushrooms, onion, tarragon, parsley, salt, and pepper, and sauté for 4 minutes, stirring occasionally.

Put in the eggs and scramble, stirring constantly, until they are prepared for about 2 minutes. To serve, divide between 4 plates.

# Grilled Fruit Salad

Preparation time: 15 minutes

Cooking time: 5 minutes

Servings: 4

Fruit doesn't always need to be raw; in reality, grilling or broiling fresh fruit brings out its natural sugars and magnifies its taste. Double the recipe and use the leftovers as a side meal for chicken or seafood.

Ingredients

8 slices fresh or canned (unsweetened) pineapple

4 fresh nectarines or peaches, pitted and sliced into 8 pieces each

8 (1/2- inch-thick) pieces fresh honeydew melon.

1 teaspoon honey, warmed for 30 seconds in microwave

1/2 teaspoon salt.

Directions:

Preheat the broiler and line a baking sheet with aluminum foil.

Spread out the fruit in a single layer on the baking sheet and brush with the honey on both sides. Spray the salt over the leading and put the pan 3 inches listed below the chicken.

Broil for 3 minutes, turn each piece of fruit, then broil for 2 minutes more, or just up until the fruit is a little browned at the edges.

Place 2 pineapple pieces, 8 peach slices, and 2 melon slices onto each of 4 plates and serve warm.

# Hearty Hot Cereal with Berries.

Preparation time: 15 minutes

Cooking time: 20 minutes

Servings: 4

Whole grains are not only terrific for your heart; they're also terrific for your waist. The high fiber material makes them filling and provides slow, constant energy for your day. The addition of berries and nuts in this dish makes it especially hearty.

Ingredients

4 cups water.

1/2 teaspoon salt.

2 cups whole rolled oats.

1/2 cup sliced walnuts.

2 teaspoons flaxseed.

2 tablespoons honey.

1/2 cup fresh blueberries.

1/2 cup fresh raspberries.

1 cup low-fat milk.

Directions:

In a medium pan, bring the water to a boil over high heat and include the salt.

Stir in the oats, walnuts, and flaxseed, then decrease the heat to low and cover.

Prepare for 16 to 20 minutes, or up until the oatmeal reaches the preferred consistency.

Divide the oatmeal between 4 deep bowls and leading each with 2 tablespoons of both blueberries and raspberries. Add 1/4 cup milk to each bowl and serve.

# Broccoli - Curry Soup

Preparation time: 20 minutes

Cooking time: 20 minutes

Serving: 4

Ingredients:

Salt & Black pepper (as needed)

Onion (1)

Curry (1 tbsp.)

Coconut oil (2 tbsp.)

Vegetable stock (1 liter)

Coconut cream (1 cup)

Sharp cheese - your choice/keto-friendly (.75 cup)

Broccoli (1 lb.)

Directions:

Pour the coconut oil into a skillet on the stovetop over a burner turned to the med-high temperature setting. Chop and sauté the onion and add to the pan for about six minutes.

Reduce the temperature to medium. Then, add in the broth until it begins to simmer. Mix in the broccoli and any seasonings before adding in the curry and letting it simmer for 20 minutes.

Pour into a blender before mixing in the cheese, and serve.

# Chicken Cauliflower Rice Soup

Preparation time: 20 minutes

Cooking time: 20 minutes

Serving: 6

Ingredients:

Carrots (2 peeled)

Celery (2 stalks)

Onion (1 small)

Chicken breast (1)

Ghee or olive oil (2 tbsp.)

Bay leaf (1)

Pepper & salt (as desired)

Fresh thyme (1 tsp.)

Chicken stock/broth (4 cups)

Canned coconut milk - full fat (2 cups)

Cauliflower rice (2 cups)

Directions:

Chop or dice the celery, carrots, and onions. Discard the skin and bones from the chicken.

Melt the ghee or pour the oil into a large soup pot. Toss the onions, celery, and carrots into the pot and cook until the veggies begin to soften (5-8 min.).

Pour in the chicken stock, bay leaf, salt, pepper, and thyme.

Once boiling, lower the heat setting to simmer. Add the whole chicken breast. Place a top on the soup pot and simmer for an additional 15-20 minutes.

Take the pan from the heat. Trash the bay leaf. Carefully take the chicken from the pot. Place on a cutting surface to shred.

Toss the shredded chicken back into the pot and simmer until it's done (5 min.).

Pour in the milk and parsley, cooking until hot and serve.

# Crockpot Chicken Chowder

Preparation time: 20 minutes

Cooking time: 20 minutes

Serving: 4

Ingredients:

Garlic clove (1)

Cilantro (1 tbsp.)

Chicken broth (1 cup)

Chicken breasts (1 lb.)

Onion (1 small)

Cream cheese (8 oz.)

Diced tomatoes (14 oz.)

Diced jalapeno (.5 oz.)

Fresh lime juice (1.6 oz.)

Salt (1 tsp.)

Black pepper (1 tbsp.)

Directions:

Remove the skin and bones from the chicken.

Chop the garlic and cilantro. Dice the onion and jalapeno.

Combine all of the fixings in the crockpot.

Prepare using the low-temperature setting for six to nine hours or high for four hours.

Once it is done, shred the chicken in the pot using two forks.

## Green Soup

Preparation time: 20 minutes

Cooking time: 0 minute

Serving: 6

Ingredients Needed for Preparation:

English cucumber (.5 cup)

Avocado (1)

Spinach leaves (2 cups)

Gluten-free vegetable broth (.25 cup)

Black pepper (to taste)

Directions:

Dice the avocado and cucumber.

Combine all of the fixings in a blender.

Toss in the fresh herbs and serve.

# Shirataki Soup

Preparation time: 15 minutes

Cooking time: 5 minutes

Serving: 2

Ingredients Needed for Preparation:

Boneless - skinless chicken thighs (2)

Chicken stock (3 cups)

Minced ginger (1 tsp.)

Minced garlic (1 clove)

Cardamom (.25 tsp.)

Mushrooms (.5 cup)

Optional: Chili sauce (1 tsp.)

Chopped cilantro (1 pinch)

Thinly sliced chili pepper (1)

Directions:

Heat the stock on the stovetop using the med-high heat setting. Toss in the ginger, garlic, mushrooms, and cardamom. Simmer for about ten minutes.

Fold in the chicken and cook until done or about five minutes.

Prepare two soup bowls and add the sliced chili pepper to each dish. Serve the soup and garnish with cilantro.

Adjust spices as desired.

# Spring Soup with a Poached Egg

Preparation time: 10 minutes

Cooking time: 5 minutes

Serving: 2

Ingredients:

Eggs (2)

Chicken broth (1 qt. - 32 oz.)

Chopped romaine lettuce (1 head)

Salt (as desired)

Directions:

Bring a pan of the chicken broth to a boil.

For a slightly runny egg, turn down the heat, and poach the two eggs in the broth for five minutes.

Remove the eggs and set aside into two serving dishes for now.

Chop the lettuce and toss into the broth. Simmer for a few minutes until slightly wilted.

Ladle the broth with the lettuce into the bowls with eggs and serve.

# Unstuffed Cabbage Roll Soup

Preparation time: 10 minutes

Cooking time: 10 minutes

Serving: 9

Ingredients:

Minced garlic cloves (2)

Small diced onion (half of 1)

80/20 Ground beef (1.5 lb.)

Bragg's Aminos (.25 cup)

Tomato sauce (8 oz. can)

Beef broth (3 cups)

Keto-friendly Worcestershire sauce/another substitute (3 tsp.)

Diced tomatoes (14 oz. can)

Chopped cabbage (1 medium)

Pepper (.5 tsp.)

Parsley (.5 tsp.)

Salt (.5 tsp.

Also Needed: Instant Pot

Directions:

Prepare the Instant Pot using the sauté mode to brown the beef, garlic, and onions. Drain and add it back to the pot with the rest of the fixings.

Set the unit on the soup function.

Natural-release the pressure of the cooker for about ten minutes. Quick-release the rest of the steam to stir and serve.

# Semifreddo Peach

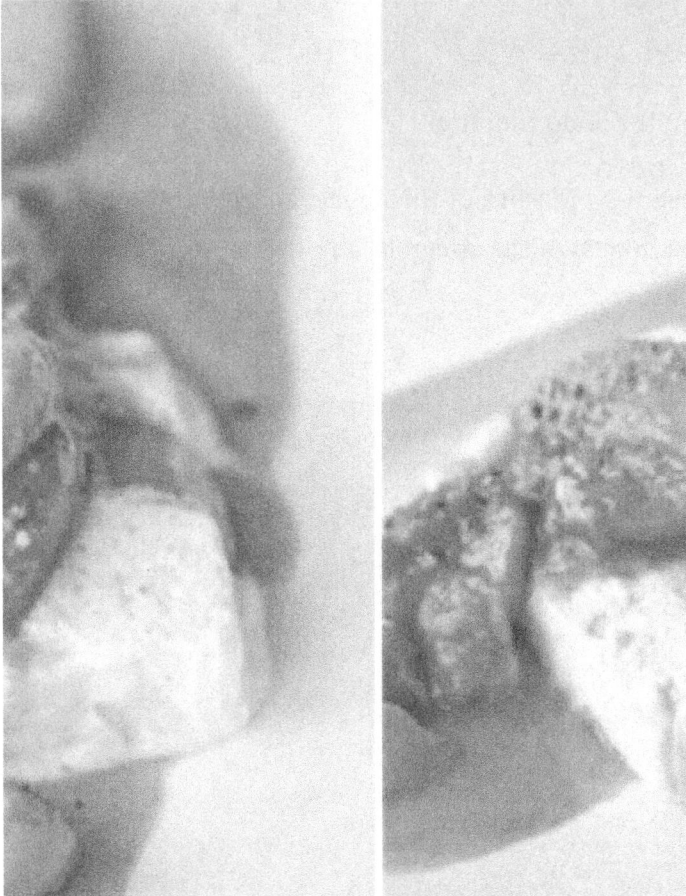

Preparation time: 10 minutes

Cooking time: 0 minute

These frozen desserts may look good, but they are also healthier than they seem. Walnuts include omega-3 fats and fibers, as well as crispy, and Greek yogurt has up to fourteen grams of protein per cup.

Servings: 4

Ingredients

4 medium peaches, sliced.

4 containers (6 ounces) of Greek vanilla yogurt.

1/2 cup of non- salted nuts, chopped

Directions:

Divide the ingredients into 4 semi-fried desserts or. Start with a layer of peaches; Then include a tablespoon of yogurt and then distribute the nuts.

# Fish rods

Preparation time: 10 minutes Cooking time: 15 minutes

Servings: 6

Ingredients:

10 ounces of tilapia fillet

½ cup coconut flour

2 beaten eggs

1 teaspoon salt

½ teaspoon ground black pepper

3 oz grated parmesan

1 teaspoon butter

Directions:

Chop the tilapia fillet and put it in the bowl. Add coconut flour, beaten eggs, salt, ground black pepper, and grated cheese. Stir the mixture with the help of the spoon until it is homogeneous. Distribute the mold generously with the butter. Put the fish mixture in the pan and flatten it well. Cut the mixture on the bars with the help of the knife. Preheat oven to 360F. Place the mold in the oven and cook the fish bars for 15 minutes or until the fish bars acquire the golden surface. Cool cooked food well and only then transfer it to serving dishes.

# Fried cod

Preparation time: 5 minutes

Cooking time: 10 minutes

Servings: 2

Ingredients:

12 ounces of cod fillet

1 tablespoon of chopped chives

1 tablespoon of butter

1 tablespoon of coconut oil

1 teaspoon of chopped garlic

1 teaspoon of cumin seed

1 teaspoon coriander seeds

1 teaspoon salt

Directions:

put the butter and coconut oil in the pan and melt them. Add garlic, cumin and coriander seeds. Rub the fish fillet with salt and put it in the pan. Fry the fish for 2 minutes on each side or until it turns light brown. Transfer the cooked cod fillet to the plate and cut it into 2 portions.

# Whole meal pancakes with blueberries and nuts

These pancakes are a delicious way to start the day. Cranberries are sour, but candies and nuts add a crunchy texture to this classic of convenience.

Preparation time: 20 minutes

Cooking time: 10 minutes

Servings: 4

Ingredients

1/2 cup fresh blueberries

3/4 cup whole wheat flour

2 tablespoons sugar

1 tablespoon of baking powder

1/4 teaspoon salt

1/2 teaspoon ground nutmeg

1/2 teaspoon pure vanilla extract

1 1/4 cup low-fat milk

1 large beaten egg

1 / 2 cups chopped walnuts

1 tablespoon coconut oil, divided

Directions:

In a small bowl, combine the blueberries with a handful of whole wheat flour, mix well to cover. In a large bowl, add the flour, sugar, baking powder, salt, and nutmeg, stirring to mix well. Add the egg, vanilla, and milk and stir to mix; however, do not mix too much. The dough should be a bit embarrassing. Carefully add the blueberries and nuts (with flour) and set the dough aside for 10 minutes. In a large, heavy skillet, heat approximately 1/2 teaspoon of coconut oil over medium heat. Pour enough dough into the pan to make a 6-inch pancake. Cook for about 2 minutes or until the edges are bright, then turn the pancake and prepare for 1 more minute. Transfer to a plate and cover overheat while preparing the rest of the pancakes. Add extra coconut oil to the pan if necessary. To serve, put 2 pancakes on each plate and cover with hot maple syrup, honey or molasses.

# Zucchini Chips

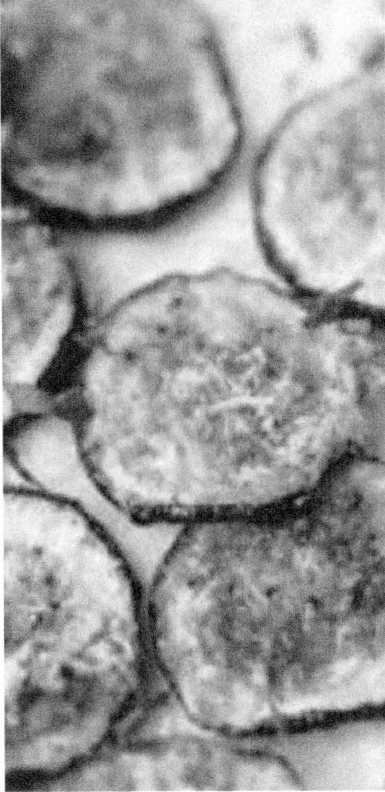

Preparation time: 10 minutes

Cooking time: 12 minutes

Servings: 4 Ingredients:

Ingredients:

1 finely chopped zucchini A pinch of sea salt Black pepper to taste 1 teaspoon dried thyme 1 egg 1 teaspoon garlic powder 1 cup almond flour

Directions:

In a bowl, beat the egg with a pinch of salt. Put the flour in another bowl and mix it with thyme, black pepper, and garlic powder. Drain the zucchini slices in the egg mixture and then in the flour. Place the french fries in a lined pan, put them in the oven at 450 ° F, and cook for 6 minutes on each side. Serve the fries as a snack.

# Pepper snack

Preparation time: 5 minutes

Cooking time: 10 minutes

Servings: 24 pieces

Ingredients:

1/3 cup of tomatoes

chopped ½ cup of peppers

mixed chopped 24 slices of peppers

½ cup of tomato sauce

4 ounces of almond cheese

diced 2 tablespoons basil

chopped black pepper

Directions:

Divide the slices of pepper on a muffin tray. Divide the pieces of tomato and pepper into the cups of peppers. Divide cubes, including tomato sauce, basil, and almonds, sprinkle the black pepper at the end, put the cups in the oven at 400 ° C, and bake for 10 minutes. Arrange the pieces of peppers in a bowl and serve. Have fun!

# Holiday meatballs

Preparation time: 10 minutes

Cooking time: 40 minutes

Servings: 20

Ingredients:

1 kg turkey ground

1 tablespoon coconut oil

melted

1 yellow onion chopped

1 egg

1 cup coconut flour

1 teaspoon Italian dressing

A pinch of sea salt

Black pepper to taste

2 tablespoons

chopped parsley

Directions:

In a bowl mix the turkey meat with half flour, a pinch of salt, black pepper, Italian seasoning, parsley, onion, egg and hot sauce and mix well. Put the rest of the flour in another bowl. Form 20 turkey meatballs and dip them in flour. Heat a pan with the oil over medium-high heat, add the meatballs, cook for 4 minutes on each side, transfer them to paper towels to remove excess fat, put them on a plate, and serve.

# Chicken fajitas

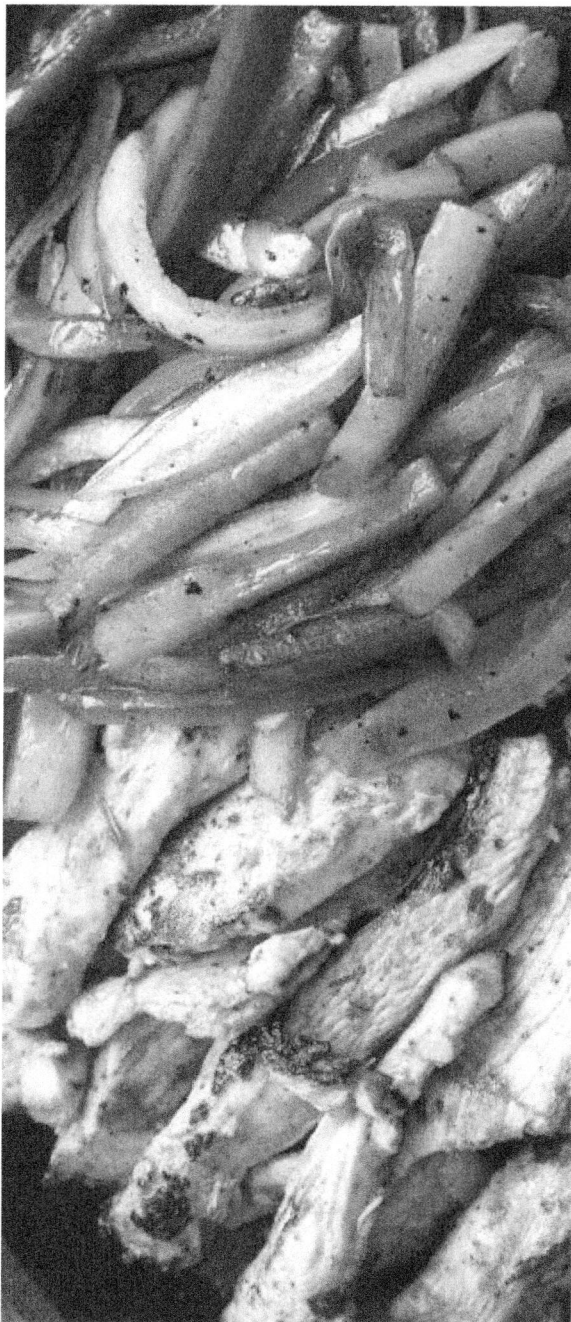

Preparation time: 10 minutes

Cooking time: 20 minutes

Servings: 4

Ingredients:

1 kilo of tender chicken

1 beaten egg A pinch of sea salt

1/3 cup of coconut

unsweetened

grated ¼ cup of coconut flour

Directions:

In a bowl, mix the coconut with the coconut flour and a pinch of sea salt and mix. Put the beaten egg in another bowl. Dip the chicken pieces in the egg, then in the coconut mixture, put them in a lined pan, and bake at 350 ° F for 25 minutes. Serve as a snack.

# Scrambled eggs with mushrooms and onions

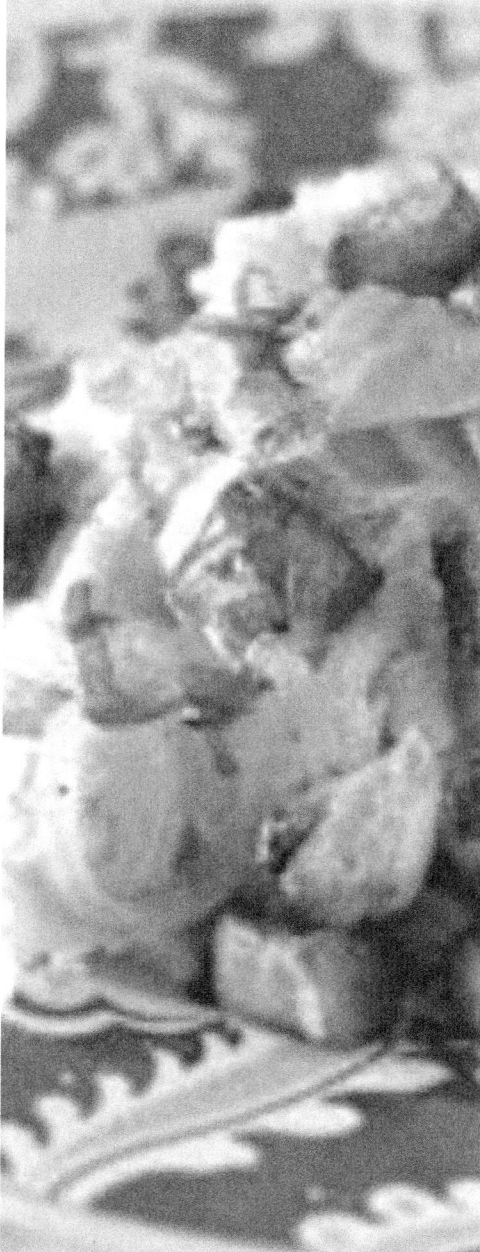

Preparation time: 10 minutes

Cooking time: 5 minutes

These eggs cook quickly, but they have a flavor that will ask you to cut and enjoy it. This also makes an excellent sandwich filling. If you need breakfast on the run, an integral pita bag is an excellent option.

Servings: 4

Ingredients:

1 teaspoon of olive oil.

1 cup sliced fresh mushrooms.

1/4 cup thinly sliced yellow onion

1 tablespoon slices of fresh tarragon.

1/2 cup chopped fresh parsley.

1/2 teaspoon salt

1/2 teaspoon freshly ground black pepper.

8 large beaten eggs.

Directions:

In a large, heavy skillet, heat olive oil over medium heat. Add the mushrooms, onion, tarragon, parsley, salt, and pepper, and fry for 4 minutes, stirring occasionally. Put the eggs and stir, constantly stirring, until they are prepared for about 2 minutes. To serve, divide by 4 dishes

# Grilled Fruit Salad

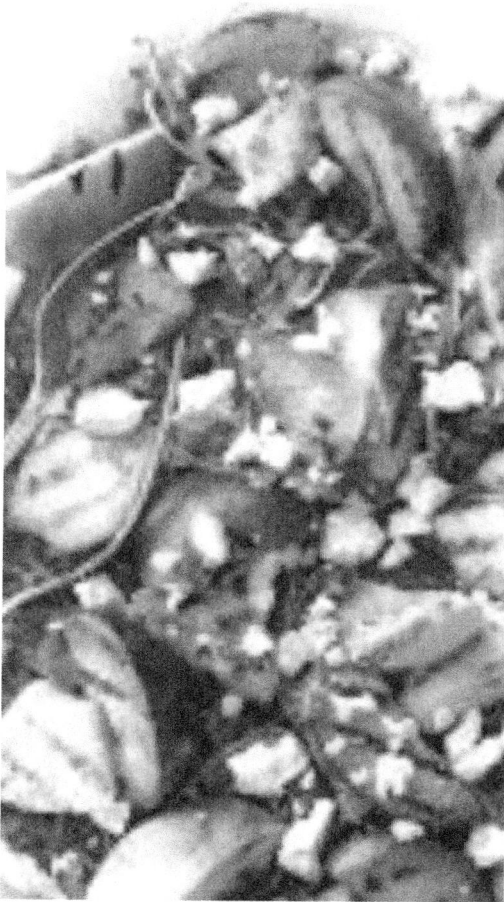

Preparation time: 15 minutes

Cooking time: 10 minutes

Fruit does not always have to be raw; In fact, toasting or roasting fresh fruit eliminates its natural sugars and increases its flavor. Duplicate the recipe and use leftovers as a side dish for chicken or seafood.

Servings: 4

Ingredients:

8 slices of fresh or canned pineapple (unsweetened)

4 fresh nectarines or peaches pitted and cut into 8 pieces each

8 pieces (1/2 inch thick) of fresh sweet melon.

1 teaspoon of honey heated for 30 seconds in the microwave

1/2 teaspoon of salt.

Directions:

Preheat the grill and cover a pan with aluminum foil. Spread the fruit in a single layer on the baking sheet and spread with honey on both sides. Sprinkle the salt on the wire and place the pan 3 inches listed under the chicken. Cook on the grill for 3 minutes, rotate each piece of fruit, then toast for another 2 minutes, or only until the fruit is lightly browned at the edges. Put 2 pieces of pineapple, 8 slices of peach and 2 slices of melon in each of the 4 dishes and serve hot.

# Abundant hot cereal with berries.

Preparation time: 20 minutes

Cooking time: 20 minutes

Whole grains are not only excellent for your heart; They are also fabulous for your life. The high fiber material fills them and provides slow and steady energy for your day. The addition of berries and nuts in this dish makes it particularly abundant.

Servings: 4

Ingredients:

4 cups of water.

1/2 teaspoon of salt

2 cups of whole oatmeal.

1/2 cup sliced walnuts.

2 teaspoons of flax seeds.

2 tablespoons honey

1/2 cup fresh blueberries.

1/2 cup of fresh raspberries

1 cup of low-fat milk.

Directions:

In a medium skillet, boil water over high heat and include salt. Add oatmeal, nuts, and flax seeds, then minimize heat and cover. Prepare for 16 to 20 minutes or until the oatmeal reaches the preferred consistency.

Divide the oatmeal between 4 deep bowls and each with 2 tablespoons of blueberries and raspberries. Add 1/4 cup of milk to each bowl and serve.

# Easy cereal bars.

Preparation time: 30 minutes

Cooking time: 40 minutes

This dish is much better for you than any industrial granola bar, which is often loaded with high-fructose corn syrup and less healthy cereals. These bars are cooked in the blink of an eye and will be kept in an airtight container for a week, that is, if they last so long.

Servings: 1 dozen of bar

Ingredients:

1 teaspoon of coconut oil.

1 cup of nut pieces

1 cup of raw pumpkin seeds.

1 cup chopped nuts.

1 cup dried cranberries.

1 cup dried apricots, sliced.

1 cup unsweetened coconut flakes.

1/4 cup melted coconut oil.

1/2 cup of almond butter

1/2 cup of raw honey

1/4 teaspoon of pure vanilla extract.

1/2 teaspoon salt

1 teaspoon cinnamon in powder.

Directions:

Preheat oven to 325 degrees F. Grease a 9-by-13-inch pan with 1 teaspoon of coconut oil and set aside. In a large bowl, combine nuts, pumpkin seeds, nuts, blueberries, apricots, and coconut flakes and mix to mix well. In a small saucepan over low heat, add melted coconut oil, almond butter, honey, vanilla, salt, and cinnamon and heat until the honey melts. Transfer the nut mixture to the pan, pushing it down to distribute evenly. Place the honey mixture evenly on top. Cook for 35 to 40 minutes or until golden brown allow the mixture to cool to room temperature before cutting into equal bars. Store in an airtight container for up to 1 week.

# Vegan Tuna Salad

Preparation time: 20 minutes

Cooking time: 0 minute

This "tuna salad" recipe includes inexpensive, easy to find ingredients that can be made in advance and stored in the refrigerator for about a week. Serve on a bed of greens, your favorite crackers, or as a classic sandwich. Feel free to add ingredients for flavor and texture, such as carrots or bell peppers.

Ingredients:

2 cans chickpeas

1 tablespoon prepared yellow mustard

2 tablespoons vegan mayonnaise

1 tablespoon jarred capers

2 tablespoons pickle relish

½ cup chopped celery

Directions:

In a medium bowl, combine chickpeas, mustard, vegan mayo, and mustard. Pulse in a food processor or mash with a potato masher until the mixture is partially smooth with some chunks.

Add the remaining ingredients to the chickpea mixture and mix until combined.

Serve immediately or refrigerate until ready to serve.

# Veggie Wrap with Apples and Spicy Hummus

Preparation time: 30 minutes

Cooking time: 0 minute

Wraps are a versatile and portable lunch option that can be adapted to any taste. The combination of the soft hummus and broccoli slaw creates a balanced texture of smoothness and crunchiness. The spicy hummus with apple brings a unique sweet and spicy blend. The end result: a lunch wrap that is anything but boring.

Ingredients:

1 tortilla of your choice: flour, corn, gluten-free, etc.

3-4 tablespoons of your favorite spicy hummus (a plain hummus mixed with salsa is good, too!)

A few leaves of your favorite leafy greens

¼ apple sliced thin

½ cup broccoli slaw (store-bought or homemade are both goods)

½ teaspoon lemon juice

2 teaspoons dairy-free, plain, unsweetened yogurt

Salt and pepper to taste

Directions:

Mix broccoli slaw with lemon juice and yogurt. Add pepper and salt to taste and mix well.

Lay tortilla flat.

Spread hummus all over the tortilla.

Lay down leafy greens on hummus.

On one half, pile broccoli slaw over lettuce. Place apples on top of the slaw.

Starting with the half with slaw and apples, roll tortilla tightly.

Cut in half if desired and enjoy!

# Mac and Cheese Bites

Preparation time: 30 minutes

Cooking time: 30 minutes

Welcome to the vegan twist on an old classic. We promised this book would help satisfy some of your old, pre-vegan cravings, so here's a great portable comfort food bite that will satisfy kids and grown-ups alike. Note that these can be eaten warm or cool, though warming them up may make them fall apart a bit.

Ingredients:

1 ½ cups uncooked macaroni (gluten-free will work if needed)

1 medium onion, chopped (can substitute with 1 medium yellow pepper if you don't care for onions.)

1 clove garlic, chopped

2 tablespoons cornstarch, or arrowroot powder

1 cup non-dairy milk

½ teaspoon smoked paprika (can substitute for chipotle powder)

1 teaspoon lemon juice or apple cider vinegar

½ cup nutritional yeast

1 teaspoon salt

Directions:

Preheat your oven to 350 degrees Fahrenheit.

Prepare the muffin tin with liners.

Prepare macaroni according to instructions.

While macaroni is cooking, sauté garlic and onion (or substitute of choice) until it is just starting to turn golden brown. This can be done in a dry pan, but adding some oil will work as well.

Add garlic, onion, and all other non-macaroni ingredients into a blender and mix until smooth.

Drain the macaroni and return to the pan.

Pour sauce over macaroni and stir well.

Spoon mixture into muffin tin, stirring occasionally in between such an equal amount of sauce goes in each cup.

Push down tops with the back of a spoon.

Bake in the oven for 30 min.

Serve once cooled.

# Chicken Salad with Cranberries and Pistachios

Preparation time: 45 minutes

Cooking time: 30 minutes

This recipe calls for soy curls (or textured vegetable protein) for the "chicken," but you could easily use tempeh or another meat substitute for choice. This salad can be served on a bed of greens, put into a wrap, or on bread as a traditional sandwich.

Ingredients:

1 ½ cups dry soy curls (textured vegetable protein)

2 dashes apple cider vinegar

½ cup diced granny smith apples (approx. 1 small apple)

¼ cup shelled pistachios, chopped

½ cup dried cranberries

5-6 tablespoons vegenaise(adjust depending on how creamy you would like the salad to be)

1 teaspoon of sea salt

A pinch of thyme

Directions:

Soak soy curls in warm water for 10 min. Squeeze excess water out of them and roughly chop larger pieces. Set aside.

While soy curls are soaking, mix diced apple and vinegar. Drain any excess liquid.

Combine apples with all other ingredients in large bowl until ingredients are evenly mixed. Add seasoning to taste. Chill for at least 30 minutes. Serve as desired.

# Mustard-Maple-Glazed Salmon.

Preparation time: 5 minutes

Cooking time: 25 minutes

Servings: 4

Ingredients

4 (6-ounce) skin-on salmon fillets, 3/4 inch thick.

1 teaspoon olive oil.

1/2 teaspoon salt.

1/2 teaspoon newly ground black pepper.

2 tablespoons pure maple syrup.

1/2 teaspoon dry mustard.

8 sprigs fresh thyme.

Directions

Preheat a flat grill over medium-high heat.

Brush the salmon fillets on both sides with the olive oil, season with salt an pepper, and place them skin side down on the grill. Cook for 7 minutes.

On the other hand, combine the maple syrup and dry mustard with a fork.

Flip the salmon fillets, brush with the maple-mustard glaze, and top each one. with 2 sprigs of the thyme. Grill for 5 to 7 minutes more, or till the fish flakes easily.

To serve, use a spatula to move the fillets to 4 plates, leaving the thyme undamaged.

# Tuscan-Style Baked Sea Bass.

Preparation time: 10 minutes

Cooking time: 20 minutes

Servings: 4

Ingredients

4 (6-ounce) skin-on sea bass fillets.

1 teaspoon olive oil.

1 cup really carefully chopped walnuts ( usage processor or blender)

2 teaspoons minced garlic.

8 pieces yellow or orange tomatoes, 1/4 inch thick.

8 slices red onion, 1/4 inch thick.

1/2 cup chopped fresh basil.

1/2 teaspoon salt.

1/4 teaspoon newly ground black pepper.

Directions

Pre-heat the oven

Brush both sides of the bass fillets with the olive oil and after that dip in the chopped walnuts, covering the fillets fully.

Place the fillets skin side down on the baking sheet. Spread the garlic over the fillets, then cover the fish with rotating tomato and onion pieces. Sprinkle the basil over the top and season with salt and pepper.

Bake for 12 to 14 minutes, or until the fish flakes quickly. To serve, use a spatula to transfer the fillets to 4 plates.

Nutrition:

Calories: 382 Cal

Fat: 16 g

Carbs: 19 g

Protein: 40 g

Fiber: 6 g

# Portobello Cheeseburgers.

Preparation time: 15 minutes

Cooking time: 20 minutes

Servings: 4

Ingredients

4 big (4 inches large) portobello mushroom caps.

1 1/2 teaspoons olive oil, divided.

1/2 teaspoon salt.

1/4 teaspoon newly ground black pepper.

1/2 teaspoon minced garlic.

1/2 teaspoon paprika.

1 cup canned cannellini beans.

4 (1-ounce) slices reduced-fat mozzarella cheese.

4 whole wheat hamburger buns.

4 big leaves romaine lettuce.

4 slices fresh tomato.

8 slices red onion.

Directions

Preheat the oven to 325 degrees F.

Rub the cap sides of the mushrooms with 1/2 teaspoon of the olive oil and season with salt and pepper.

In a big frying pan, heat the remaining 1 teaspoon olive oil over medium-high heat. Include the mushrooms, cap side down, and sauté for 4 minutes.

On the other hand, mix together the garlic, paprika, and beans and heat in the microwave for 1 minute, or simply up until warm. Set aside.

Turn the mushrooms and location 1 piece of mozzarella onto each one.

 Lower the heat to low.

Toast the hamburger buns in the oven for 5 minutes, or simply till crisp.

Transfer to 4 plates. Top the bottom buns with the tomato, onion, and lettuce.

Spoon one-quarter of the bean mixture into a mound in the center of each bun and top with a mushroom, cap side up. Add the top buns and serve.

Nutrition:

Calories: 278 Cal

Fat: 9.9 g

Carbs: 33.7 g

Protein: 9.3 g

Fiber: 2.4 g

# Conclusion

This book has shed light on the basics of intermittent fasting. It has everything that you need to know to kick start your weight loss journey. We have also provided a step-by-step guide to take you through the process.

Besides losing weight, we have emphasized the benefits that come with intermittent fasting. Even if you are not after losing weight, trying this new way of life will reward you with fantastic health in general. Besides, if you are new to intermittent fasting, we have various tips and tricks to get you going on the fast to ensure that you will encounter no complications and have a good time.

You have also learned about the things that may affect your success while fasting. We have busted many misconceptions that people hold on to in the name of fasting, as well as highlighted the healthy foods that you can consume while fasting as well.

One of the best things about intermittent fasting is that it comes in various forms, and you do not necessarily have to have to follow a particular schedule. This is why it matters to listen to your body as you go along the fast.

All in all, never forget the importance of staying hydrated while you are fasting. It can mean the difference between a smooth and tough fast. It may even help you come up with a reasonable exercise plan that will be perfect for your fasting method.

Fasting can be physically and mentally demanding. Many hurdles may make you want to throw in the towel along the way. Don't worry; this is normal. However, never lose sight of your goal. Failing one or two times is neither a crime nor a license to abandon the entire lifestyle. Allow your motivation to keep you going when it gets tough.

Before making dietary changes, it is always best to consult with a qualified healthcare professional, even if you just change the timing when you eat food. They can help you figure out if intermittent fasting would be good for you. This is particularly important for long-term fasts where there may be vitamin and mineral depletion. It's important to understand how incredibly smart our bodies are. The body will increase appetite and the number of calories consumed at the next meal if food is limited at one meal, and even slow down the metabolism to match calorie consumption. Further, intermittent fasting has many potential health benefits, but it should not be concluded that, if strictly followed, huge weight loss is assured, and disease creation or progression avoided. It is a useful tool, but it may require other tools to help achieve and maintain optimal health.

Congratulations on saying NO to ill health, stubborn weight gain, depression, dementia and premature ageing, and a loud NO to the idea that we cannot naturally heal our bodies and minds! When I first sat down to write this guide to understand and use the secrets of intermittent fasting, to people like you: those who are not satisfied with the current state of affairs, which they had been told and did not do that. They are ready to let go of their desire for good health, vitality, physical fitness, clarity of mind and longevity just because conventional medicine and nutrition tells them that this is impossible. Continuing your journey to achieve liveliness and well-being for life, remember that you are travelling through an old, proven form of prosperity. I urge you to use this as a guide. When people ask about the use of intermittent fasting, you will not only be able to point to visible changes in your body, appearance and energy levels, but you have all the scientific evidence at hand to prove that the old method works! Live and heal! These days it works just as well as centuries ago! Finally, I wish you all the best on your journey to restore, rejuvenate and protect every cell in your body and mind. This is handy for use with different types of intermittent fasting, which we cover in this guide! Good luck and good health!

Printed in Great Britain
by Amazon